INFORMATION SEARCHING In Health Care

Renee M. Williams, PT, MHSc
Lynda M. Baker, RN, MLS
Joanne Gard Marshall, MLS, MHSc, PhD

SLACK Incorporated, 6900 Grove Road, Thorofare, NJ 08086

SLACK International Book Distributors

In Japan
  Igaku-Shoin, Ltd.
  Tokyo International P.O. Box 5063
  1-28-36 Hongo, Bunkyo-Ku
  Tokyo 113
  Japan

In Canada
  McGraw-Hill Ryerson Limited
  300 Water Street
  Whitby, Ontario
  L1N 9B6
  Canada

In all other regions throughout the world, SLACK professional reference books are available through offices and affiliates of McGraw-Hill, Inc. For the name and address of the office serving your area, please correspond to

  McGraw-Hill, Inc.
  Medical Publishing Group
  Attn: International Marketing Director
  1221 Avenue of the Americas —28th Floor
  New York, NY 10020
  (212)-512-3955 (phone)
  (212)-512-4717 (fax)

Executive Editor: Cheryl D. Willoughby
Publisher: Harry C. Benson

Editorial, Production and Design Services: SHEPHERD, Inc.

Printed in the United States of America

Library of Congress Catalog Card Number: 88-43543

ISBN: 1-55642-093-5

Published by: SLACK Incorporated
               6900 Grove Road
               Thorofare, NJ 08086-9447

Contents

Chapter 2
The Resources: Putting Them to Work   49

Linking Information Searching Resources to Practice
Lynda M. Baker

Chapter 3
Critical Appraisal: Analyzing the Information 89
Linking Research to Practice
Renee Williams

Preface

The rapid increase in health care knowledge in recent years has made it essential for health professionals to have effective information searching and critical appraisal skills. These skills include the ability to find, evaluate, and apply information from the health sciences literature to health care problems. This book is intended as a guide for health professionals who want to learn these skills so that they can make the most effective use of information resources available to them.

Although this book represents a renewed and expanded effort for each of the authors, the ideas in the book and its use as a teaching tool have a longer history. We all have been involved in the education programs at McMaster University, Faculty of Health Sciences. The problem based approach to learning in the Faculty of Health Sciences puts particular emphasis on information gathering as a basis for tutorial discussion and problem solving by students. Faculty members recognize that health care knowledge changes rapidly and that the continuing competence of graduates will depend upon the skills that they develop for lifelong learning. Providing students with an opportunity to learn effective information searching and critical appraisal skills is recognized as an important basic educational objective.

This book will assist health practitioners in keeping up to date with the ever increasing amount of published health care information. The book is for all health professionals whether they are students, practitioners, educators, researchers, or administrators. Librarians and students in library and information science, who are becoming increasingly involved in the teaching of information searching skills to health professionals, will also find the work valuable. The book is appropriate as a textbook and reference work for use in both formal and informal library orientation, critical appraisal and research instruction for health care students and staff.

The authors acknowledge the assistance of Don Baker of Baker/ Moffatt Design Group, Incorporated for his expertise in the preparation of the figures and tables in the book.

About The Authors

RENEE M. WILLIAMS PT, MHSc, is assistant professor, School of Occupational Therapy and Physiotherapy, Faculty of Health Sciences and Chair of the Bachelor of Health Sciences Programme, McMaster University and research consultant, Hamilton Civic Hospitals, Henderson General Division, Hamilton, Ontario. She received a Master of Health Sciences (Health Care Practice) degree from McMaster University. Her education research interests are in evaluating the various instruments that are used to assess student learning. Her clinical research interests are in low musculoskeletal work-related injuries and the measurement of clinical instruments used in physical therapy.

LYNDA M. BAKER RN, MLS, is currently pursuing studies in the doctoral program at the School of Library and Information Science, University of Western Ontario, London, Ontario. At the time of writing, she was the Head of Reference, Health Sciences Library, McMaster University, Hamilton, Ontario. Her area of research interest is physician-patient communications and the information needs and information-seeking behavior of health care clients.

JOANNE GARD MARSHALL MLS, MHSc, PhD, is assistant professor at the Faculty of Library and Information Science at the University of Toronto where she teaches courses in Health Sciences Information Resources, Online Information Retrieval and Management of Corporate and Other Specialized Information Centres. She has had over 15 years of experience as a health sciences librarian, including several years as a clinical librarian providing information to health professionals, patients and families in inpatient and outpatient settings.

Introduction

One of the most challenging aspects of health care practice today involves trying to keep up-to-date with the ever increasing body of health care knowledge. The roots of the health professional's information dilemma are the same as those for the scientific community as a whole. Since World War II, the scientific literature and the number of researchers have both grown at exponential rates. This phenomenon is commonly referred to as the information explosion. While it is difficult to determine exactly when this phrase came into common use, many authors cite a classic article written in 1945 by Vannevar Bush, in which he noted the difficulties he experienced as a scientist trying to keep up with the findings and conclusions of thousands of other workers.[1]

In the health care field, a study of the literature on schistosomiasis, a disease caused by an infestation of the body by schistosoma, or blood flukes in infected water, provides an illustration of the information explosion in our own domain. The authors found in reviewing the literature over a 110 year period that only three percent of the literature was produced in the first fifty years, while 40 percent appeared in the last ten years.[2] Some critics argue that the information explosion cannot be equated with a similar size increase in our actual knowledge base. But, as the previously cited study also found, the ratio between total published papers and those of quality has remained constant with time. Thus, health professionals who want to keep up to date are faced with an increasing amount of literature to scan and evaluate.

The purpose of this book is to provide both students and practicing health professionals with a solid grounding in information search skills, including the critical appraisal of research evidence. Locating and evaluating information are important components of effective information use. Chapter 1 of the book presents a model for information use by health professionals and discusses the general principles of information searching. An understanding of information use patterns and the search process will provide the reader with a framework through which the nature and purpose of specific information resources can be understood. Chapter 2 describes methods of accessing the basic types of information resources, and the content and use of specific information tools in detail. This chapter is useful as a directory of information sources and can be referred to on an ongoing basis. Chapter 3 focuses on the critical appraisal of research evidence located through the information search process. This chapter presents some patient management problems, provides examples of computerized literature searches on the topics, and applies the critical appraisal process to the retrieved literature.

References

1. Bush V: As we may think. Atlantic Monthly 176:101-108, 1945.
2. Warren KS, Goffman W: The ecology of the medical literature. Am J Med Sci 263:267-273, 1972.

1

The Process: Knowing How to Start

*Linking Information Searching
Process to Practice*

Joanne Gard Marshall

Learning Objectives

After completing this chapter, the reader will be able to:

- Recognize information searching as a method of keeping up to date with constantly changing health care knowledge;
- Discuss the information needs and information seeking habits of health professionals;
- Describe a model for using information from the health sciences literature in patient care;
- Recall the broad categories of information resources in the health sciences;
- Compare methods of locating books and journal articles through print and electronic sources;
- Design an information search strategy based on an analysis of the concepts presented in a health care problem;
- Describe specific search strategies for retrieving journal articles that meet critical appraisal criteria; and
- Practice the ethical and professional use of information resources, including appropriate citing of sources, observation of copyright law and use of required bibliographic style in papers and publications.

Building a Professional Knowledge Base

A professional knowledge base is the body of knowledge and experience that a health professional draws upon every day to make decisions. The value of the professional within the health care system depends largely upon the existence of this knowledge base and the individual's demonstrated ability to solve clinical, educational, administrative and research problems. Students begin acquiring a knowledge base through classes, course work and hands on experience in patient care settings. Educational programs are designed to provide students with the level of knowledge that they need to start functioning at a professional level. But, as any practitioner knows, the knowledge gained as a student is only the beginning of a continuing process of lifelong professional learning. This opportunity for continuous learning is one of the major factors that makes a career in the health professions stimulating and challenging.

Maizell has estimated in the technical fields that the half life of what a scientist or engineer knows is close to ten years.[1] Half of what the technical professional has learned will be obsolete in a decade, and half of what the professional will need to know in ten years is not available now. As a result, professionals must constantly update and increase their knowledge base using methods such as work experience, discussions with colleagues, reading the literature and attending conferences. Taking an active role in developing and improving your knowledge base is part of what it means to be a professional. For health professionals, the consequences of failing to maintain an adequate knowledge base may involve individual sanctions by professional regulatory groups and even the loss of the right to practice. The maintenance of a sound professional knowledge base is just as important in the areas of administration and research as it is in clinical practice. Effective information seeking skills are required to accomplish the ongoing task of building and maintaining a professional knowledge base. These skills are used by health professionals to fill knowledge gaps and to keep up to date with new developments.

Information Needs of Health Professionals

An understanding of the information needs of health professionals and how these needs are best met can assist in analyzing and improving your own information seeking habits. One way of gaining this insight is to examine previous research findings. Based on a series of interviews with scientists and science reference librarians, Voigt proposed a useful classification system for scientific information needs based on three approaches: the current approach, the everyday approach and the exhaustive approach.[2] This system suggests that scientists have three types of information needs:

1. To keep up with new or current information;
2. To find specific pieces of existing information related to the work that must be accomplished on a daily basis; and
3. To do a comprehensive search of all the existing research that has been done on a particular topic.

As Voigt points out, keeping up with one's subject field is mandatory for all active scientists. The methods that scientists commonly use to meet their current information needs include: conversing with colleagues and visitors, attending conferences and meetings, corresponding with others working in the same field; reading the scientific literature, using indexes and abstracts, reading review articles and reading monographs, i.e. books on a single subject. Health professionals often use general journals received as part of professional memberships with organizations such as the American Nurses Association, the American Occupational Therapy Association or the American Medical Association and browse among the current journals in a health sciences library as a means of meeting their current information needs.

The everyday approach is taken when information directly related to one's daily work is required. An example of a nurse's every day information need might be to interpret an abbreviation found on a patient's chart, an occupational therapist might need more information about a self help device, or a social worker might need information about respite care facilities available in the community for Alzheimer's disease patients and their families. Conversations with colleagues are an important means of meeting everyday information needs, although a variety of other sources, including handbooks or directories, may also be required. Everyday information needs are often met through a single piece of information such as a name, address or brief description, but they can also require a search of the recent literature for appropriate readings on a subject.

Voigt's exhaustive approach is taken when a full search of the literature is required. This type of approach is much less frequent than the current or everyday approaches previously described; taking the exhaustive approach usually means that a major project is underway. Perhaps a health professional is considering applying for a research grant and needs to know what previous related research has been done. Or perhaps a health professional is making an educational presentation to colleagues on a topic and he or she is expected to be the expert on the subject. At various times, health professionals will use each of these approaches to meet their information needs.

A research project at McMaster University found that the majority of information needs in health care settings tend to be of the everyday variety, or at least they start out that way.[3] Some everyday information needs relate to the confirmation of existing knowledge to ensure that nothing has changed since the orginal information was acquired. In other cases, unsolved problems in work settings generate the need for new information. These problems become the subjects of discussions with colleagues and searches of the health care literature, e.g. perhaps a health care team cannot find an adequate instrument for the functional assessment of a particular type of patient and a search is begun.

When a literature search is undertaken, practitioners most frequently want a few recent references that are directly related to a specific topic, e.g. the use of home defibrillators for high risk cardiac patients. Sometimes these patient care questions develop into major research ideas or interests. Perhaps there are no clinical trials found on the use of defibrillators at home and a properly designed study needs to be done. If this is the case, a more comprehensive approach to information searching is required before a final decision about initiating the study is taken. Similar findings about the origins of information needs in patient care settings to those discussed here were reported in a study at the University of New Mexico.[4]

The McMaster study cited earlier found some additional frequent information needs.[3] Journal articles or other works reviewing the state of the art on a given therapy or disease were used extensively by students and new staff members from the various health professions as a means of acquainting themselves with the topic or updating their basic knowledge. Physicians, in particular, requested information from another specialty in situations where a patient had multiple problems, e.g. an obstetrician treating a pregnant lupus patient asked for recent articles on the medical treatment of lupus.

Members of the allied health professions often requested information on certain aspects of care, at least partially as a means of demonstrating the importance of some of their concerns to their colleagues on the health care team, e.g. a nutritionist asked for journal articles on the relationship between diet and osteoporosis, a social worker requested information about the possible depressive side effects of a drug and a nurse asked for some articles on improving the functioning of health care teams. The latter nursing example illustrates that the information needs of health professionals frequently relate to administrative and organizational issues as well as to direct patient care. The increasing emphasis on measurement of quality of health care, including medical audit, peer review, and utilization review, create many new information needs for health professionals. Clinical librarians at University of California at Los Angeles (UCLA) cancer treatment center found that they were responding to two main types of physician information needs.

1. To locate information on correctly diagnosing and treating a rare or unusual problem; and
2. To determine whether there was so little literature on a patient care problem that a published account of their own experience of it should be made.[5]

The latter information need points out that information seeking activities, especially those that are research related, are not always initiated with the expectation of finding information on a topic. Sometimes, not finding something is just as important or more important than finding the information. Not finding something points to a gap in the health care knowledge base which may serve as the impetus for a research project or a report of clinical findings. A summary of the reasons for information searching health care that have been discussed in the preceding section is provided in Table 1-1.

In the context of meeting everyday information needs, the information search becomes a dynamic and purposeful activity for health professionals. Not only do the results of the information search assist in solving a particular health care problem, but they also contribute to the

Table 1-1. Summary of Reasons for Health Care Information Searching

1. To confirm of disconfirm existing knowledge.
2. To assist in solving a new or unfamiliar health care problem.
3. To update basic knowledge on a topic through a state-of-the-art review.
4. To obtain information from another specialty when dealing with a patient with multiple problems.
5. To highlight particular patient care concerns to other members of the health care team.
6. To find out about a rare or unusual patient care problem.
7. To determine whether a knowledge gap exists in the literature and whether a new research project or publication should be planned.
8. To assist in implementing new administrative or organizational initiatives such as quality assurance programs.

maintenance and enhancement of the searcher's professional knowledge base. As Dykes states, "adults learn best what they have to know to modify their performance and tend to forget information that they do not use."[6] He urges health professionals to look for facts that are clinically relevant, to separate them from facts that are not, and to keep the latter in the background to be retrieved as needed. This approach can be very helpful in coping with the sheer amount of information available on a given health care topic. One need not read and absorb all of the information found. Instead, one should use a scanning mode to look for the particular piece of information that will help to make a judgment about the problem at hand.

Information Seeking Habits of Health Professionals

While many health professionals believe that they have developed adequate information seeking skills, there is considerable research evidence to show that both practitioners and researchers tend to under utilize formal information sources such as books and journals.[7-10] Other studies have shown that libraries and librarians have not been highly valued by clinicians, even though they can provide access to a broad and authoritative body of information.[11-12] Friedlander found that researchers working in theoretical fields were more likely to use formal information sources such as libraries, whereas professionals in applied fields, such as engineering and medicine, were more likely to use informal sources such as colleagues.[11] Reliance on informal sources of information was found to be especially strong in the health sciences, more so than in other areas of science. Rubenstein found that researchers consulted formal written sources more often than clinicians, but neither were found to make frequent use of librarians.[12]

In the health field, sources of information about drugs constitute a special problem because many of the most easily accessible sources, e.g. pharmaceutical representatives and printed drug information provided by pharmaceutical companies, are also the least objective. Herman and Rodowskas, Jr. reported that physicians mentioned commercial sources 4.7 times as frequently as independent professional sources for learning about new drugs. The major sources of drug information for American Medical Association members were *Physicians' Desk Reference* and opinions of colleagues. Fifty-two per cent of the respondents named pharmaceutical representatives as their major sources of drug information.[13]

Leaving aside for the time being the particular problem of drug information, one question that needs to be asked is whether there is anything really wrong with relying upon people rather than books and journals for information. There are many advantages to consulting another person as opposed to a book or journal article and, as Voigt's research showed, scientists frequently do use other people as a primary information source for dealing with everyday information needs.[2] Another person can listen to you express your information need in your own words and will frequently help you to refine your question. A knowledgeable colleague can often help you to ask the right question rather than pursuing a time consuming and fruitless information searching course. Often, colleagues can provide you with an opinion or judgment based on a synthesis of their own knowledge and experience.

In a study of scientific information channels, Thomas found that there was more reliance on word of mouth for the transmission of scientific data than previously reported and that the system seemed to function with reasonable accuracy and reliability.[14] Crane has written about the phenomenon of informal information exchange among scientists and called it the "invisible college."[15] This invisible college of colleagues near and far forms an essential part of the information seeking world of scientists. Shibutani, in a classic sociological work, actually defends the integrity of rumor in everyday life by stating that rumor that takes place through critical deliberation is often cross checked for plausibility and reliability of sources.[16] This type of rumor often represents the informal pooling of expert knowledge. Most of us would readily admit that we rely to a considerable extent on what we hear from others and find it reliable enough to meet many of our information needs.

In the health care field, however, Greene brings some words of caution about the limitations and pitfalls associated with verbal communication alone as a means of acquiring accurate information.[17] Greene provides examples of situations in which false information was verbally transmitted along with accurate information. He points out that there are established controls over the quality of information published in books and refereed journals through peer review, while there are no such documented assurances about the contents of informal conversations.

Some medical authors suggest that verbal communication is the best, and sometimes the only, way to find the latest research findings on a particular topic.[7,14] But they also argue that basic knowledge in a subject area and the results of authoritative studies are best gleaned from formal sources such as books and journals. Greene suggests that it is unwise to accept gossip or verbal opinion as the sole basis for decision making in any instance regarding patient care decisions.[17]

Recent research shows that health professionals typically gather information from at least three different sources prior to making a change in their practice behavior.[18] For instance, a health professional might attend a conference and hear a paper on a new therapy or technique, then check it out through some recent journal articles in the library and finally, discuss it with colleagues in their department before deciding to use it. This system of using multiple methods of information gathering and confirmation appears to be the most responsible approach for health professionals to take in developing their own information seeking habits. A number of different studies have shown that journals are still the most frequently cited source of information by health professionals.[19-20] These findings reinforce the need for health professionals to be knowledgeable about the use of many of the information resources discussed in this book.

A Model for Information Seeking in Health Care

Given what we know from the previous review of information needs of health professionals, building a good set of information seeking habits based initially on the everyday approach mentioned in Voigt's classification makes a lot of sense.[2] Figure 1-1 presents a model that includes various aspects of the dissemination and use of information in health care settings based upon observations from one of the earlier cited studies.[3]

As Figure 1-1 indicates, health professionals are frequently presented with problems in their **work situation** that require more information before a decision can be made. Perhaps a decision is required about recommending home apnea monitoring devices to parents whose infants are at risk for Sudden Infant Death Syndrome. Questions from patients about new therapies that they have read about in a newspaper or magazine may require further investigation before a health professional can give an informed opinion. The introduction of new management techniques or standards of care in health care settings may require additional information before implementation decisions can be made. A certain level of discipline is required to use these everyday situations as opportunities for continuing learning. At busy times it is easy to let such opportunities slip by without follow up or to act on the basis of past experience. The first good habit to develop is one of prompting oneself and others to ask questions. This stage is referred to as **question generation** in Figure 1-1. For example, if a patient is experiencing difficulty coping with the side effects of therapy, are there other treat-

Figure 1-1. A Model for Information Seeking In Health Care

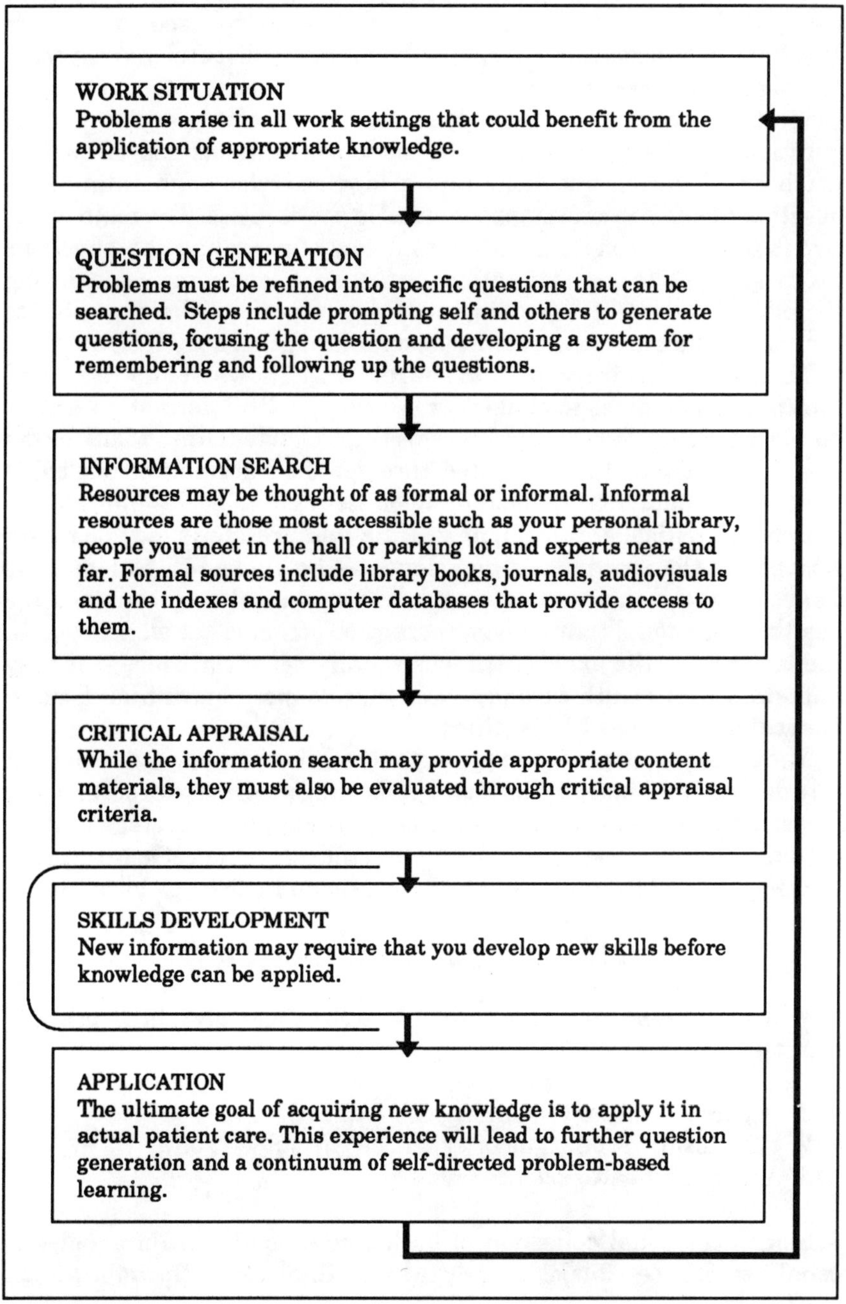

WORK SITUATION
Problems arise in all work settings that could benefit from the application of appropriate knowledge.

QUESTION GENERATION
Problems must be refined into specific questions that can be searched. Steps include prompting self and others to generate questions, focusing the question and developing a system for remembering and following up the questions.

INFORMATION SEARCH
Resources may be thought of as formal or informal. Informal resources are those most accessible such as your personal library, people you meet in the hall or parking lot and experts near and far. Formal sources include library books, journals, audiovisuals and the indexes and computer databases that provide access to them.

CRITICAL APPRAISAL
While the information search may provide appropriate content materials, they must also be evaluated through critical appraisal criteria.

SKILLS DEVELOPMENT
New information may require that you develop new skills before knowledge can be applied.

APPLICATION
The ultimate goal of acquiring new knowledge is to apply it in actual patient care. This experience will lead to further question generation and a continuum of self-directed problem-based learning.

ments that should be considered that do not have the same side effects? Is there recently published evidence of the effectiveness of the treatment being used? This kind of mental questioning can be used to generate questions for information seeking or during group discussions that occur at rounds and other clinical activities. As a series of questions is generated, have a notebook handy or other means of keeping track of the questions so that a record can be made of them. Instead of using a notebook, dictating questions into a tape recorder or maintaining a question file on a microcomputer are also possibilities. The main objective is to have a convenient, habitual way of recording the questions before going on to the next patient or task. Set some time aside during the day or the week, depending upon the urgency of the situation, to reconsider the questions and decide on information search strategies.

The steps in the **information search** stage shown in Figure 1-1 and the specific resources available for locating health information will be discussed in detail in Chapter 2 of this book. **Critical appraisal,** or the evaluation of the studies located through the information search, is covered in Chapter 3. Depending upon the results of the information search and critical appraisal, new **skills development** may be necessary before the new idea or technique can be applied to patient care. Conversely, the information search and appraisal may convince the health professional that a given therapy or action is not warranted. In the latter case, the exploration was equally beneficial since it is very important that health care practices that do more harm than good in particular situations be identified.

The ultimate purpose of acquiring information is to apply it to patient care decision making, as illustrated in the final **application** stage of the model. Far from being the end of a process, the application stage is likely to lead to further question generation and the continuum of learning that is needed to maintain an effective professional knowledge base.

The Information Search

When beginning an information search, there are three possible starting points:

1. A personal library or information file;
2. Consulting a colleague or expert on the subject; or
3. Visiting a health sciences library.

Since a personal collection of books, notes and journal articles is usually most accessible, it is likely to be the first stop on the information

search route. Readers who need some advice on developing a personal
filing system are referred to publications by McCarthy and Haynes et
al.[22-23] Figure 1-2 illustrates the types of information resources that may
be available and the various search paths that can be taken.

Figure 1-2. Information Search Path

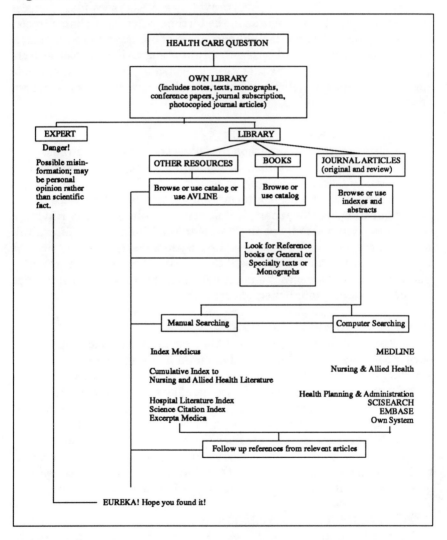

Another way of organizing document categories suggested by Stibic can be used to think about different kinds of information resources.[24] Primary literature consists of books, journal articles, dissertations, reports and other types of documents. Works which provide means of accessing the primary literature are considered to be secondary sources. Secondary sources include bibliographies, catalogs and indexing and abstracting services. A third level providing access to secondary sources is referred to as tertiary. Works in the tertiary category include directories of information services, bibliographies of bibliographies and directories of computerized databases. Before starting an information search, there are several questions that deserve consideration. The answers to these questions are helpful in selecting the most appropriate search route and information resources.

1. *From where are you starting?*

Are you a novice or an expert on the subject or somewhere in between? Novices are advised to obtain some basic information from a textbook or review article before consulting an expert or the latest research literature on the topic. The basic information will prepare the novice to ask better questions of the expert, if that route is selected later. Having a basic background also helps the novice to read the research literature more knowledgeably. The more expertise you have, the more likely it is that the information you need will come from other experts or recently published journal articles. You may even need to track down conference proceedings and unpublished papers.

2. *What do you want to know?*

How much of an expert do you want to become on this topic? Consider an earlier search example from this chapter on home apnea monitoring. Do you simply want to know what equipment is required, in which case a description from a health care device handbook might suffice, or do you need to know about the controversies surrounding this type of monitoring? Would you like to read a few recent articles on etiology and incidence of Sudden Infant Death Syndrome? Perhaps the hospital has a major concern about the advisability of home apnea monitoring and you have been asked to do a comprehensive review of the literature. These are the type of questions that must be asked in order to define your information need.

3. *What resources are available to you?*

All health professionals do not have the same level of access to information resources. Some health professionals have built up excellent personal libraries over time that meet many of their information needs. Others have access to departmental collections of textbooks and core journals. Most hospitals have a library of some type, but the level of staffing, collection and services generally deped upon the extent of teaching and research in the institution and the level of support from the hospital administration.

Health sciences libraries in the United States have access to a Regional Medical Library Network which facilitates the borrowing and lending of materials among libraries. In Canada there are also a number of formal and informal hospital library networks in operation. Some health professionals practice in academic settings with large libraries that support research, education and patient care. The ease with which these various levels of resources are available to health professionals clearly affects information searching capabilities. Fortunately, the computer age is making it easier for health professionals outside of major centers to access a wide range of information resources. Inquire with your nearest health sciences librarian about what can be accessed in your locale and how you can best take advantage of the resources.

4. *How much time and money do you have to spend?*

Information searching is often time consuming, which means that it can also be expensive if the value of the individual's time is taken into account. An additional expense may be incurred if online databases are searched. Charges for database access are made by online search services and these are usually paid by the institution or the individual health professional requesting the search. Many libraries are now subscribing to CD-ROM databases which may lower costs substantially. A recent letter to the *New England Journal of Medicine* suggested that database searches for patient care should be reimbursed by programs such as Medicare and Medicaid.[25] Database searches are usually very cost beneficial because the equivalent manual search of the indexes and abstracts would be much more time consuming. Nevertheless, the cost benefit of searching activities should be evaluated in relation to the value of the information required and received. The next part of this chapter is devoted to looking at the characteristics and uses of various types of formal information resources such as books, journals, computer databases and other learning materials. Although these resources are discussed primarily in the library context, the comments apply equally to the same type of materials in your own personal collection.

Types of Information Resources

Reference Books

Books can be categorized on the basis of the purpose for which they are used. A reference book is usually consulted for a single item of information rather than being read from cover to cover. Typically, reference books include directories, dictionaries, encyclopedias and handbooks of various sorts. Examples of the kind of information found in a reference book include the address of a colleague (directory), the definition of a syndrome (dictionary), short treatises on a topic (encyclopedia) and normal lab values (handbook). In a library, reference books are usually kept in a conveniently located, separate section for quick consultation, just as one might keep a dictionary on a desk in an office. Because they are frequently used, reference books are usually restricted to use within the library.

Textbooks

Textbooks are an important resource because they represent core knowledge. Students and practitioners study from textbooks; they also use the most recent edition of textbooks as the first place to look for basic information. Because textbooks are often consulted for single items of information, they can also be considered a kind of basic reference book. Texts such as the *Lippincott Manual of Nursing Practice, Harrison's Textbook of Internal Medicine, Medical-Surgical Nursing,* and *Conn's Current Therapy* are published in new editions frequently. *Scientific American Medicine* is published under a continuous revision arrangement where the subscriber periodically receives updates to different sections. But, even with these frequent publication schedules, textbooks are at least partially out of date when they are published because of the preparation time involved. Textbooks have also been criticized on the basis that they often present expert opinion rather than the evidence upon which the opinions are based.

Despite these limitations, textbooks, both general and specialty, are a good starting place for the novice searcher or for a health professional who needs a quick refresher on a topic before launching into a more extensive search. Textbooks are used so often in health sciences libraries that they may be kept in a separate section and the loan period may be shorter than for other books in the collection. Although you may want to keep a few key texts in your personal library, the expense of keeping up with the latest edition will likely prove difficult. Rely on the closest hospital or health sciences library for these sources.

Monographs

Books that treat a single topic in depth are often referred to as monographs. Like textbooks, monographs suffer in terms of currency because of the time required for their preparation and publication. Nevertheless many monographs are considered to be classic works providing the most comprehensive discussion of a subject. A personal collection may well include a few selected monographs related to the owner's specific interests or area of expertise.

Annual Reviews and Other Collected Works

This group of publications falls between the book and journal categories. Like books, annual reviews and collected works can be in depth works on a single theme or subject. As the name suggests, however, annual reviews are published every year. Collected works, which may serve a similar purpose to the annual review, are published on a one time, or irregular, basis. Annual reviews and collected works usually consist of a number of papers by different experts and reflect the state of the art in a given field. Because the contents reflect experts' perceptions of important new developments in the field, practitioners often use annual reviews as a way of meeting current information needs.

These types of publications are sometimes difficult to track down in a library because of their "in between" nature. Many health sciences libraries put their books in one section of the library and their journals in another. Annual reviews are usually indexed by the journal indexes and may be shelved with the journals in the library. However, if the annual review or collected work has monographic qualities, i.e. if it is more of an in depth treatise on a single topic than a collection of miscellaneous papers, it may be cataloged as a book. It is difficult to state hard and fast rules about the handling of these types of publications, but consult a librarian if in doubt about how to find them in the library.

Journals

Last of the types of information resources on the list, but definitely not least, is the journal. Journals are also referred to as periodicals or serials. Books are usually published as single works, whereas journals are published periodically, or serially, as the synonyms imply. Journals can be issued weekly, monthly, or at any other regular interval. The term "magazine" is usually applied to popular periodicals or serials, such as *Time* magazine, and the term "journal" is preferred for scientific and professional publications, such as the *Journal of Applied Psychology* and the *American Journal of Occupational Therapy*. Journals are the primary publication type in any scientific library, constituting about 70 percent of the volumes in the collection.

Currency

Why are journals so important in the health sciences? A major reason is the currency of the information they contain. Authors can write a journal article more quickly than an entire book and the publication schedules of journals are usually more rapid than those for books. But in recent years even the journals have been criticized for not being up to date. Some journals take up to two or more years to publish an article after it is accepted for publication. To acknowledge the date of the original work, many journals now routinely print the date of submission of the original manuscript and the date of acceptance of the paper in the journal. Despite criticisms about publication delay, journals are still considered to be the most up to date source of authoritative scientific information.

Peer Review

Another major reason for the primacy of the journal literature in science is the process of peer review. Following an initial screening by the editor, articles submitted to "refereed" journals are usually sent to a minimum of two expert reviewers for comments and a judgment about whether the article should be published. A journal's rejection rate is viewed by some to be a measure of journal quality. The peer review process is generally considered to be the most effective way of guaranteeing trustworthy scientific information. Book manuscripts also undergo a form of editorial and peer review. But, in the sciences especially, the review process for books generally is not seen as being as competitive and demanding as the review process for journal articles.

Journal Article Format

A standard format has developed for the journal article that reflects its primary purpose as a reporting vehicle for scientific research findings.[26] It begins with an abstract, i.e. a short summary of the contents and findings reported in the body of the article. The first section of the article provides background to the research, including the purpose and research questions. A review of the literature on the topic is included in the introductory section so that the study is linked to previous important work. A section on data gathering and research methods includes details of sampling, the approach taken to data analysis and the statistical measures used. The results section is usually followed by a discussion in which the author elaborates on the implications of his or her findings. Data summaries are often presented in numeric form as tables interspersed in the text. Highly efficient systems for indexing and abstracting the journal literature have developed over the years. The existence of these access tools undoubtedly has encouraged and sustained the frequent use of journal articles as a medium for scientific communication. The searching of these indexes and abstracts in print and electronic forms will be discussed in detail later in this chapter.

Other Resources

A variety of audiovisual media and computer assisted instructional packages are used today by health professionals as mediums for basic learning and continuing education. However, books and journals remain the most frequently used forms of research communication in the health sciences. These printed sources are portable, browsable, can be read on the subway, train or bus and are nice to curl up with in the evening. For these reasons, book and journal resources have been stressed in this chapter.

Finding Books

The Library Catalog

In a personal library it may be sufficient to organize books alphabetically by author or to group them by general subject. But in a library, because of the numbers of books involved, the system has to be more elaborate. Libraries store the information about the books in their collection in a **catalog.** Until recently, most library catalogs were in card form and the books could be looked up in the card catalog under the author(s), the title of the book, or the subject(s) covered in the book. A set of cards was produced by the library for each book and the cards were filed under a variety of access points to allow users to find the listing for the book. Today, many libraries are computerizing their cataloging system. Once the catalog records are in "machine readable form," a variety of catalog formats are possible. A library might have a computer produced printed catalog or perhaps use computer output microfiche (COM) or microfilm. Some libraries have online public access catalogs (OPAC) that allow the user to search the catalog using a computer terminal in the library. Large libraries may even allow access to the library catalog from remote locations elsewhere in the building or the local area. No matter what format is used for the catalog, the basic principles described earlier about catalogs making the collection available under a variety of access points still applies. Find out what system your library uses and how to use it most efficiently.

Call Numbers

Why do health professionals use a library catalog? Often the catalog is used to find out if the library has a particular book. In this case, the fastest way to look up the book is by author or title. Alternatively, subject headings may be looked up to find out what books the library has on a specific topic. Once the book is found in the catalog, the user will likely want to locate the book on the shelf in the library. For this purpose, the user needs to make a note of the call number.

What is a **call number?** A call number is a unique combination of letters and numbers assigned to a book that can be used as a locating device. For instance, the call number for a book entitled *Thinking Through Writing* by Susan R. Horton is PE1408.H6836. The call numbers are placed on the spine of the book in the following way:

PE
1408
.H6836

To find this book in the library, first look for the **PE** section and then follow the numerical arrangement until the volume is located on the shelf. The assigning of call numbers to books is based on a **classification system.** Most classification systems organize the information resources in the library into some type of general subject arrangement. If you are familiar with the classification system used by your library, this knowledge of the broad subject classification can be used to browse the collection. For instance, if the user knows that books on pediatrics are found in the WS section, he or she might decide to go straight to the shelves and browse through the pediatric books rather than using the catalog.

Although health professionals frequently use browsing as a method of looking for books in the library, there are some limitations to this approach that should be kept in mind. Books, in particular, are often on loan from the library, so the user may be missing some of the most important works. In addition, a classification number can place a book in only one place on the shelf. For instance, if a book deals with nutrition and the elderly, the cataloger will classify it under either nutrition or elderly depending on which concept is considered to be the dominant one in the book. In the catalog, on the other hand, subject headings would be given for both nutrition and elderly. In general, browsing should only be used when a very casual approach to information retrieval is considered sufficient.

Classification Systems

The most commonly used classification systems in health sciences libraries are the National Library of Medicine (NLM) classification scheme and the Library of Congress (LC) scheme. The call number notation for these two systems follows a similar format using a combination of letters and numbers. Libraries that use NLM classification for medical and related preclinical sciences also use LC classification for nonmedical subjects, such as religion, philosophy, psychology and sociology. If a library uses NLM classification, the medical books will be found under the letter *W*. If a library uses LC for its medical books, they will be found under the letter *R*. Because LC is a general classification system which covers all areas of knowledge, it takes a more limited approach to detailed classification in specific medical subject areas. NLM's mandate, on the other hand, is to develop a specific classification system for the medical sciences. NLM is usually the classification system of choice in hospital libraries and other specialized medical collections. LC is often used in academic libraries where the health sciences library may be part of a more general university library system. Health sciences libraries frequently use LC classification for nonmedical books in their collections. This works out very well since the two systems have been designed to be compatible.

Outlines of the two classification schemes follow in Figure 1-3 and Tables 1-2 to 1-3. Two versions of the NLM classification scheme are provided, one based on the subject structure and the second presented as an alphabetized list of the subjects with initial call letters. It is interesting to look at the subject structures in classification schemes just to get an idea of how knowledge is organized in a discipline.

Finding Journal Articles

The importance of journal literature in the health sciences was discussed at length earlier in this chapter. Most information searches conducted in the library will include a search for journal articles. The library catalog alerts you to the existence of books on a subject and often to the titles of periodicals held by the library as well, e.g. *Pediatric Clinics of North America*. What the catalog does not do is tell the user of the existence of specific articles within journals on particular topics. To find out about specific articles, it is necessary to use the separately published indexes and abstracts. These access tools for journal literature are usually located adjacent to the reference books in the library. In any case, they will be in a central location in the library because they are used frequently. In health sciences libraries the journals are usually shelved separately from the books and arranged alphabetically by the title of the journal. The *List of Journals Indexed in Index Medicus* is most often used as a guide to the alphabetic arrangement. The alternative practice for libraries is to assign call numbers to journals like those given to books and to shelve the journals in subject classified order. The advantage of the alphabetic arrangement is that the user does not need to obtain a call number to find a journal on the shelf. Of course, the alphabetic arrangement does not allow for any kind of grouping according to subject. Find out which of these methods for shelving journals is used by your library before looking for journals.

Figure 1-3. Library of Congress Classification Schedules

LIBRARY OF CONGRESS CLASSIFICATION SCHEDULES

A	General Works
B-BJ	Philosophy, Psychology
BL-BX	Religion
C	Auxiliary Sciences of History
D	History: General and Old World (Eastern Hemisphere)
E-F	History: America (Western Hemisphere)
G	Geography, Maps, Anthropology, Recreation
H	Social Sciences
J	Political Science
K	Law (General)
KD	Law of the United Kingdom and Ireland
KE	Law of Canada
KF	Law of the United States
L	Education
M	Music
N	Fine Arts
P-PA	General Philology and Linguistics, Classical Languages and Literatures
PA Supplement	Byzantine and Modern Greek Literature, Medieval and Modern Latin Literature
PB-PH	Modern European Languages
PG	Russian Literature
PJ PM	Languages and Literatures of Asia, Africa, Oceania, American Indian Languages, Artificial Languages
P-PM Supplement	Index to Languages and Dialects
PN, PR, PS, PZ	General Literature, English and American Literature, Fiction in English, Juvenile Belles Lettres
PQ Part I	French Literature
PQ Part 2	Italian, Spanish, and Portuguese Literatures
PT Part I	German Literature
PT Part 2	Dutch and Scandinavian Literatures
Q	Science
R	Medicine
S	Agriculture
T	Technology
U	Military Science
V	Naval Science
Z	Bibliography, Library Science

Table 1-2. Synopsis of Classes

NATIONAL LIBRARY OF MEDICINE

SYNOPSIS OF CLASSES
(Book Call Numbers)

PRECLINICAL SCIENCES

QS	Human anatomy	QW	Microbiology and Immunology
QT	Physiology	QX	Parasitology
QU	Biochemistry	QY	Clinical Pathology
QV	Pharmacology	QZ	Pathology

MEDICINE AND RELATED SUBJECTS

W	Medical Profession	WK	Endocrine System
WA	Public Health	WL	Nervous System
WB	Practice of Medicine	WM	Psychiatry
WC	Infectious Diseases	WN	Radiology
WD 100	Deficiency Diseases	WO	Surgery
WD 200	Metabolic Diseases	WP	Gynecology
WD 300	Diseases of Allergy	WQ	Obstetrics
WD 400	Animal Poisoning	WR	Dermatology
WD 500	Plant Poisoning	WS	Pediatrics
WD 600	Diseases by Physical Agents	WT	Geriatrics, Chronic Disease
WD 700	Aviation and Space Medicine	WU	Dentistry, Oral Surgery
WE	Musculoskeletal System	WV	Otorhinolaryngology
WG	Cardiovascular System	WW	Ophthalmology
WH	Hemic and Lymphatic Systems	WX	Hospitals
WI	Gastrointestinal System	WY	Nursing
WJ	Urogenital System	WZ	History of Medicine

Indexes and Abstracts

A **periodical index** generally provides author and subject access to articles contained in the important journals in the field. In preparing the index, the professional indexer has looked at the journal article, recorded the basic bibliographic information and provided a number of subject headings that describe the content. Some commonly used health sciences indexes include *Index Medicus, International Nursing Index, Cumulative Index to Nursing and Allied Health Literature (CINAHL), Index to Dental Literature* and *Hospital Literature Index.*

An **abstract**, by contrast, contains both the indexing information and a short summary of the contents of the article. A distinction usually is made between publications that reproduce the author abstract, i.e. the abstract that the author(s) prepared for publication with the article in

Table 1-3. Classification in Subject Order

THE NATIONAL LIBRARY OF MEDICINE
CLASSIFICATION SCHEME

GENERAL BOOK SUBJECTS
in alphabetical order

PRECLINICAL SCIENCES. MEDICINE AND RELATED SUBJECTS

Anatomy (Human) QS	Metabolic Diseases WD 200
Animal Poisoning WD 400	Musculoskeletal SystemWE
Aviation and Space Medicine WD 700	Nervous System WL
Biochemistry QU	Nursing WY
Cardiovascular System WG	Obstetrics WQ
Clinical Pathology QY	Ophthalmology WW
Deficiency Diseases WD 100	Otorhinolaryngology WV
Dentistry and Oral Surgery WU	Parasitology QY
Dermatology WR	Pathology QZ
Diseases of Allergy WD 300	Pediatrics WS
Diseases of Physical Agents WD 600	Pharmacology QV
Endocrine System WK	Physiology QT
Gastrointestinal System Wl	Plant Poisoning WD 500
Geriatrics, Chronic Diseases WT	Practice of Medicine WB
Gynecology WP	Psychiatry WM
Hemic and Lymphatic Systems WH	Public Health WA
History of Medicine WZ	Radiology WN
Hospitals WX	Respiratory System WF
Infectious Diseases WG	Surgery WO
Microbiology and Immunology QW	Urogenital System WJ
Medical Profession W	

the journal and other sources that write their own original abstracts. As might be expected, there are more indexes than abstracts available because indexes are less time consuming and costly to prepare. However, abstracts can be extremely useful because of the additional information they provide about the contents of the journal article. Some commonly used abstract publications in the health sciences include *Excerpta Medica, Abstracts of Hospital Management Studies, Biological Abstracts* and *Psychological Abstracts.*

The journal articles appear in the periodical indexes and abstracts anywhere from two months to two years after they are published. The particular indexes and abstracts often have policies for assigning priority to the indexing of certain journals. In any case, a journal issue that arrived in the library the previous week will not yet be accessible through the indexes. For this reason, if the very latest information is required, the user should scan the journal shelves in the library. There is a publication called *Current Contents* that reproduces the title pages of journals and provides an index to keywords in the title of the article. *Current Contents* is published weekly and is concurrent with the publication of the journal issues. When using any of these indexing and abstracting tools, find out what journals are covered by them. Most of the indexes and abstracts publish a list of journals indexed. Perhaps there are key journals from a field that are not included in the more general indexes and these articles will be missed if this is not recognized. For instance, there are a number of family medicine journals that are not included in *Index Medicus,* but another index called *FAMLI (Family Medicine Literature Index)* has very comprehensive coverage of international family practice literature. There is a very useful publication called *Ulrich's Periodicals Directory* which lists where journals are indexed. The major indexes and abstracts usually are available in printed form in the library. However, many of these useful tools are also available in electronic form as computer searchable databases. Understanding how to use the printed indexes and abstracts provides an excellent basis upon which to evaluate and use the electronic versions.

Searching Tips

When preparing a list of references, whether they are from the catalog or the indexes and abstracts, it is an excellent idea to use 3 x 5 inch cards or slips of paper. Once the items are recorded on the cards, they can be sorted in whatever order is most useful for the task at hand. For instance, the cards could be sorted by call number when looking for books on the shelf and by journal title when looking for journals (assuming that your library organizes journals in this way). This procedure can save a lot of running back and forth in the library looking for different items. If some books or journal issues cannot be located on the shelves, keep the cards in a separate group and make further inquiries at the Circulation Desk in the library. When it is time to write a paper, the cards can be arranged in the order in which they are cited in the paper or in alphabetical order by author, depending upon the bibliographic style being followed. At the end of this process, the cards can be added to a personal information file.

Another useful tip is to make sure to write down complete references for each book or journal article on the card. In the case of books, this includes the author(s), title, edition (if other than the first), place of publication, publisher and date of publication. For journal articles you will want the author(s), title, name of the journal, year, volume number, issue number, and first and last pages of the article. Since this information is needed to cite the source properly in a paper, taking down the complete information when it is first found can save a lot of return trips to the library to track down missing parts of citations. Sample book and journal citations are shown in Figures 1-4 and 1-5.

Figure 1-4. Sample Book Reference

SAMPLE BOOK REFERENCE

Bemier, Charles L. and Yerkey, A. Neil.
Cogent Communication: Overcoming Reading Overload.
Westport. Conn: Greenwood Press, 1979.

Call no: HM 258
    .B47

Figure 1-5. Sample Journal Reference

SAMPLE JOURNAL REFERENCE

Strother EA, Lancaster DM, Gardiner J.
Information needs of practicing dentists.
Bull Med Libr Assoc 1986 Jul; 74(3):227-230.
Source of reference: Index Medicus

Database Searching

Since the production of indexes and abstracts is an ongoing, labor intensive task, publishers are constantly seeking new ways of producing these tools more quickly and efficiently. In the mid-sixties, some of the major publishers, including the National Library of Medicine, began to use computers to produce their indexes. Computers were used to sort and format the indexed material and were seen initially as labor saving devices in the publication process. Once this information was in machine readable form, however, computer programs were also developed to search the indexes electronically as online databases.

In 1988 there were almost 4,000 online databases available and over 500 online search services.[27] A **database** is defined as a collection of data or information, usually with a common subject theme. Publicly accessible databases are available through commercial online search services such as DIALOG and BRS. Online search services typically provide online search service contracts, as well as providing training and support for database users. A list of some of the major online search services is provided in Table 1-4.

The term "online" indicates that a database is searched in an interactive mode via telecommunications lines. The searcher requires a data terminal or a microcomputer with telecommunications software and a modem. A modem is a device that allows electronic signals to be sent and received via telephone. The searcher dials a local telecommunications

Table 1-4. List of Major Online Search Services

LIST OF MAJOR ONLINE SEARCH SERVICES

BRS Information Technologies
A Division of Maxwell Online
8000 Westpark Drive
McLean,VA 22102
1-800-289-4277

Dialog and Knowledge Index	
In Canada: Micromedia Limited	In US: Dialog Information Services, Inc.
158 Pearl Street	Marketing Department
Toronto, Ontario MSH IL3	3460 Hillview Avenue
416-593-5211	Palo Alto, CA 94304
1-800-387-2689 (Toll Free)	1-800-3-DIALOG

ORBIT Search Service
A Division of Maxwell Online
8000 Westpark Drive
McLean, VA 22102
1-800-456-7248

MEDLARS (NLM)	
In Canada: Health Sciences Resource Centre	In US: National Library of Medicine
Canada Institute for Scientific and Technical	8600 Rockville Pike
Information	Bethesda, MD 20894
National Research Council	1-800-638-8480
Ottawa, Ontario K1A OS2	
613-993-1604	

PaperChase
Longwood Galleria
350 Longwood Ave.
Boston, MA 02115
617-732-4800

network, enters the numeric address for the online search service, and then signs on to the service with a user number and password. Once signed on, the appropriate database is selected and the search is conducted.

MEDLARS

The National Library of Medicine (NLM) provides an online search service for the MEDLARS databases which it also produces. **MEDLARS** stands for **MED**ical Literature **A**nalysis and **R**etrieval **S**ystem, an acronym used to describe the entire computerized retrieval system of NLM. There are over twenty different MEDLARS databases that provide access to over 9.5 million references to the world's professional literature in the health sciences. Databases in the health sciences are among the most established and comprehensive of any subject field. Some of the most frequently searched databases include MEDLINE (the electronic version of *Index Medicus, International Nursing Index,* and *Index to Dental Literature*), and Health Planning and Administration (the electronic version of *Hospital Literature Index*). Another frequently used database is Nursing and Allied Health (the electronic version of *Cumulative Index to Nursing and Allied Health Literature),* available through DIALOG. One of the most useful features of the MEDLINE and some of the other databases is that they contain author abstracts for a substantial proportion of articles in the databases which are not available in the printed indexes. A list of the major MEDLARS databases is shown in Table 1-5.

Table 1-5. Selected List of MEDLARS Databases

DATABASE	PRINTED PUBLICATION(S)	COVERAGE
AIDSLINE	No separate print publication	1980–
AVLINE	NLM Audiovisual Catalog	1975–
BIOETHICSLINE	Bibliography of Bioethics	1973–
CANCERLIT	No separate print publication	1963–
CATLINE	NLM Current Catalog	1801–
HEALTH PLANNING & ADMINISTRATION	Hospital Literature Index	1975–
HISTLINE	Bibliography of the History of Medicine	1964–
MEDLINE	Abridged Index Medicus, Index Medicus, Index to Dental Literature, International Nursing Index	1966–
SDILINE	Current month of MEDLINE	

SELECTED LIST OF MEDLARS DATABASES

Full Text Databases

The most frequently searched databases in the health sciences are still what are called "bibliographic" databases, i.e. those that contain the author, title, source and sometimes an abstract of an original article. But there are increasing numbers of full text databases becoming available. These full text databases contain the source document in its entirety. Examples of full text databases in the health field include *Comprehensive Core Medical Library, Drug Information Full Text* and *Consumer Drug Information Full Text*.

End User Searching

Until recently, most online searches were conducted by search intermediaries located in libraries and information centers. Now a number of the online search services are developing and marketing simplified "end user" systems to encourage health professionals to conduct their own online searches using a microcomputer at home or in the office. Some libraries have also made end user searching available in the reference department. These end user systems usually provide the searcher with a series of choices from menus, whereas experienced intermediaries use command language to tell the computer what to do. The wide array of online systems and databases makes it confusing for the health professional to decide which system to use, but some guidance is provided in the literature.[28,29]

One of the most popular ways for end users to access the NLM databases is by using a software program called *Grateful Med*. This reasonably priced program allows the user to enter the computer search "offline", i.e. before connecting to the online service. Once the search strategy has been entered, the user instructs the program to proceed. *Grateful Med* then automatically signs on to the NLM computer in Bethesda, Maryland, performs the search and transfers or downloads the results to the user's own microcomputer disk. Considerable cost savings result from using *Grateful Med*, particularly for novice searchers. Yet another search option has been developed by some large academic health sciences libraries that have made MEDLINE, or a subset of MEDLINE, available as part of the same local electronic information system as their online catalog. Johns Hopkins has an information system called Welmed that includes access to MEDLINE 500. Georgetown University has developed miniMEDLINE, and at UCLA there is a Melvyl MEDLINE. In these systems, users are presented with a menu of databases that includes the library catalog, MEDLINE and, in some cases, other databases as well. These advanced systems suggest that the libraries of the future will likely be libraries of electronic databases, as well as libraries of books and journals.

CD-ROM

The most recent technology for electronic database storage is CD-ROM, a short form for Compact Disc-Read Only Memory. This new mass storage medium allows up to 275,000 pages of text to be stored on a single 4.7 inch silver disc. One disc holds one year of the full MEDLINE database or several years of a more limited subset of the journals indexed in MEDLINE. CD-ROM discs are accessed through a microcomputer with an attached CD-ROM drive. When speaking of computer storage discs, the type of discs that are read only, such as CD-ROM, is usually spelled "disc." Computer discs on which users can both read and write their own information, as in word processing, are spelled "disk." Electronic systems of the future will likely make use of both types of disks for different purposes.

The advantage of CD-ROM is that the user is not being charged for online use of the database. However, the cost of the reader and the MEDLINE CD-ROM subscriptions is substantial. *The Cumulative Index to Nursing and Allied Health Literature (CINAHL)* also has become available recently in CD-ROM format from a company called SilverPlatter. Health sciences libraries that conduct frequent database searches for their users and other hospital departments with specialized information needs, such as the emergency department and the drug information service, are starting to subscribe to CD-ROM products. Other new kinds of mass information storage devices will be available in the future. Research on end users of online databases shows that there is considerable variability in the way that health professionals use online databases. Both frequency of use and skill levels vary.[30] If health professionals require only one or two searches a month, they are wise to continue delegating online searches to trained search intermediaries such as librarians. Even health professionals who decide to do some of their own searching often continue to delegate more complex and comprehensive searches to trained search intermediaries. A health professional's decision about using online database and end user searching will depend to a great extent upon the resources available in their own environment. But database searching no doubt will play an increasingly important part in the information seeking activities of health professionals in the future.

Designing an Information Search Strategy

Whether one is starting a search by using the library catalog, printed indexes and abstracts, computer databases, or a combination of these information seeking tools, the first step in designing an information search strategy is to define the search question. Let's take a practical example:

A 70 year old patient has recently arrived on the ward with a diagnosis of Parkinsonism. Although there are a number of different aspects to the situation, you initially are interested in finding out what drug therapies have been used successfully in the elderly. What are the major concepts in this question? Certainly the question has to do with Parkinsonism but, in this case, with a particular aspect of treatment, it also has to do with drug therapy. Even if recent articles on drug treatment for Parkinsonism were located, they probably would not completely satisfy your information need, because you really want to know what treatments are suitable for the older patient. Thus, there appear to be two major concepts in this search:

1. Parkinsonism (drug therapy); and
2. Elderly.

This approach to analyzing a search question and breaking it down into component concepts is called the building blocks approach in the information science literature.[31] Using this technique can be very helpful in clarifying a question, identifying the key elements in the information search and specifying the relationship between the concepts involved in the search. The concept map shown in Figure 1-6 is a useful guide for preparing a search strategy.

Once the major concepts in a search question are identified, the next step is to evaluate the concepts. Are the concepts of equal importance? If we can look under only one of the concepts to start the search, is one concept more important than the other? Is one concept more specific than another? When using a printed index, it is a good idea to start searching under the most specific concept first because you will have to look through fewer references to find the right articles. In database searching, we have the luxury of being able to combine the various concepts in the search. Nevertheless, it is still a good idea to begin with the most important concept. In the Parkinsonism search example cited above, the disease name appears to be the best starting point. What now?

Using MeSH

One could try going straight to the *Index Medicus* with the search concept in mind. However, there is an important step to take before going to the index. The National Library of Medicine has developed a list of subject terms called *Medical Subject Headings* (MeSH). *MeSH* lists the authorized terms that are used by NLM to catalog books and to index

Figure 1-6. Search Strategy Concept Map

SEARCH STRATEGY CONCEPT MAP

Concept A	(AND)	Concept B	(AND)	Concept C

(OR)

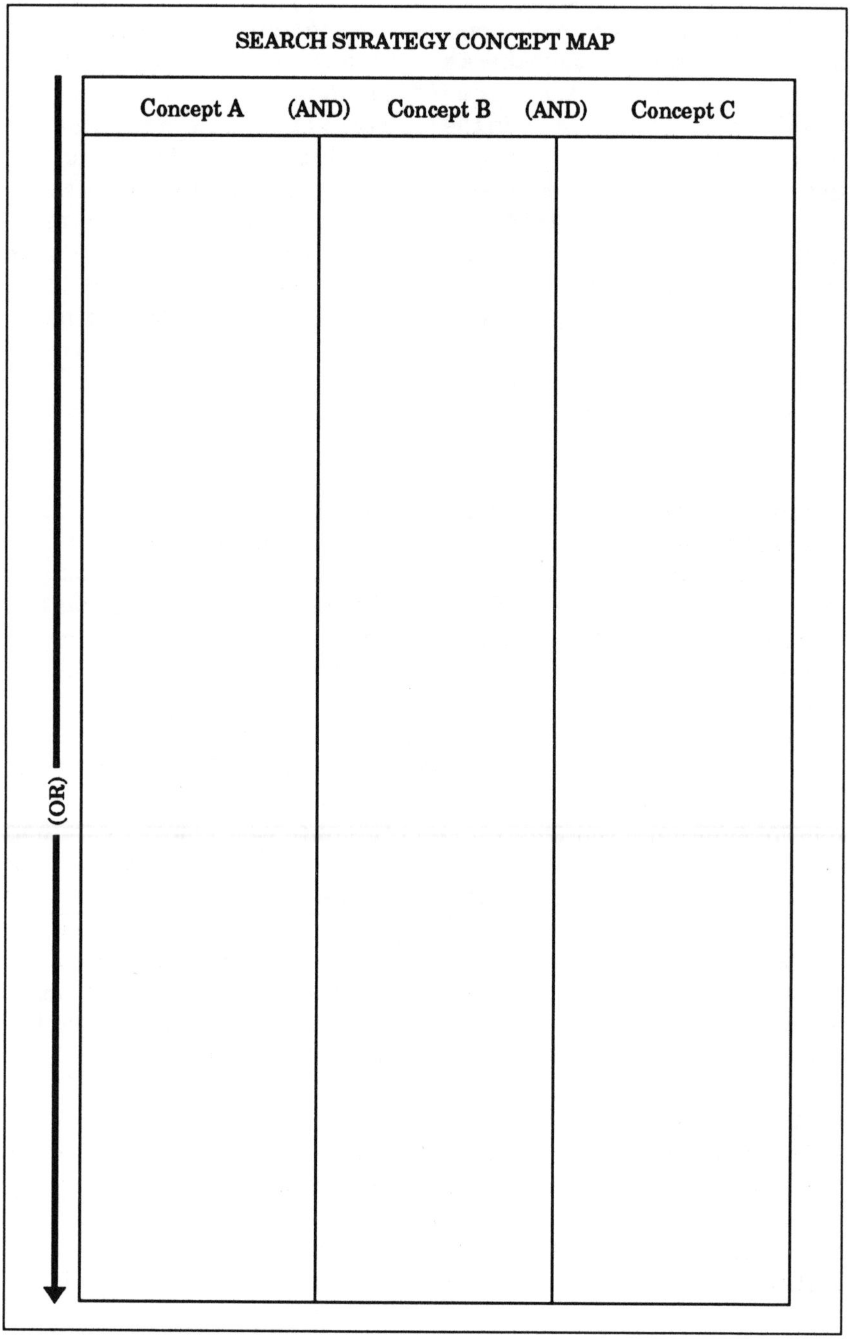

journal articles. An updated version of *MeSH is* published annually and issued with the January issue of *Index Medicus.*

There are many advantages to using terms from *MeSH* in information searches. The most important advantage is that, in *MeSH,* a single term or phrase has been used to represent a particular concept, such as Holistic Health, Patient Discharge, or Parenteral Hyperalimentation, no matter how it was referred to in the original title or abstract of an article. For the *MeSH* examples just given, other wording, such as alternative medicine, discharge planning, or parenteral nutrition, might well have been used by the authors in their works on the subject. Given the variability in authors' use of language, having standard *MeSH* terms assigned to publications is a great advantage.

Our own search example is a case in point. When we look up the term that was initially used to describe the disease, Parkinsonism, in *MeSH* the term is not listed in that form. Instead, there are three terms which appears as follows:

1. PARKINSON DISEASE;
2. PARKINSON DISEASE, POSTENCEPHALITIC; AND
3. PARKINSON DISEASE, SYMPTOMATIC

Clearly, Parkinsonism is not the indexers' authorized way of referring to the disease, even though it is sometimes used in everyday language. The entry for Parkinson Disease found in *MeSH* is shown in Table 1-6.

A close examination of the notes under the the PARKINSON DISEASE entry in *MeSH* reveals that we should also consider using ANTIPARKINSON AGENTS. Since we want drug therapy of Parkinsonism, this latter term looks most appropriate, but it is still not time to look up some journal articles in the index. Let's look under ANTIPARKINSON AGENTS in *MeSH* as shown in Table 1-7. Here we find the history of the use of ANTIPARKINSON AGENTS as an indexing term, including when it was first introduced. *MeSH* follows changes in health care knowledge and language usage and this, in turn, affects search strategies for different time periods.

Under the term ANTIPARKINSON AGENTS there is an alphanumeric code: D14.307+. So far we have been using the Alphabetic Section of *MeSH* but, if we look up this code in another section of *MeSH,* we will find an entire list of specific drugs that are used to treat PARKINSON DISEASE. The section in the back of *MeSH is* called the **Tree Structures** because it presents the *MeSH* terms in a hierarchy from general to specific. The Tree Structures can be visualized as a kind of tree of subject terms. The branches actually divide and subdivide, like a real tree, into smaller and smaller units. The Trees can be browsed up and down to

Table 1-6. MeSH Entry for PARKINSON DISEASE

MeSH ENTRY FOR PARKINSON DISEASE

PARKINSON DISEASE
  C10.228.140.79.804+ /drug ther: consider also ANTIPARKINSON AGENTS; /chem
  ind=PARKINSON DISEASE, SYMPTOMATIC/chem ind
  79; was PARKINSONISM 1967-78, was PARALYSIS AGITANS 1963-66
  use PARKINSON DISEASE to search PARKINSONISM & PARALYSIS
  AGITANS back thru 1966
  X PARALYSIS AGITANS

PARKINSON DISEASE, POSTENCEPHALITIC
  C10.228.140.79.804.832.751 C10.228.140.437.238.739
  79; was PARKINSONISM, POSTENCEPHALITIC 1967-78
  use PARKINSON DISEASE, POSTENCEPHALITIC to search
  PARKINSONISM, POSTENCEPHALITIC back thru 1967

  see related
  ENCEPHALITIS, EPIDEMIC
  X POSTENCEPHALITIC PARKINSONISM

PARKINSON DISEASE, SYMPTOMATIC
  C10.228.140.79.804.832+
  /chem ind permitted: coord IM with drug/ad-poi-tox (IM); coord IM
  with other cause (IM)
  79; was PARKINSONISM, SYMPTOMATIC 1973-78
  use PARKINSON DISEASE, SYMPTOMATIC to search PARKINSONISM,
  SYMPTOMATIC back thru 1973
  X PARKINSONIAN SYNDROME

PARKINSONIAN SYNDROME see PARKINSON DISEASE, SYMPTOMATIC
C10.228.140.79.804.832+

---

locate both more general and more specific *MeSH* terms related to the
term with which we started.

Note that ANTIPARKINSON AGENTS comes under the more general
category of CENTRAL NERVOUS SYSTEM DEPRESSANTS, one of the
bigger branches on the tree.

This presents something of a dilemma. Do we have to look under all
of the drug names separately? In the *Index Medicus,* general articles on
ANTIPARKINSON AGENTS would be found under that term, but articles
on a drug like LEVODOPA would be indexed under the more specific drug
name. The golden rule of indexing is to always index under the most
specific term available. Perhaps a look in *Index Medicus* under AN-
TIPARKINSON AGENTS would be enough to satisfy our information need
and provide us with one or two general review articles. If not, then it is
probably time to consider a database search.

There is a special capability available on MEDLINE, the computerized
version of *Index Medicus,* which allows us to "explode" a category of

Table 1-7. MeSH Entry for ANTIPARKINSON AGENTS

```
            MeSH ENTRY FOR ANTIPARKINSON AGENTS

ANTIPARKINSON AGENTS              Tree number indicating that more
D14.307+ ──────────────────       specific terms exist

76; was ANTIPARKINSON DRUGS 1973-75,
was ANTIPARKINSON DRUGS see under
PARASYMPATHOLYTICS 1963-72
XR PARASYMPATHOLYTICS ──────  There is a cross reference from
                              parasympatholytics, a related term

                              The heading can be found under four
                            ╱ more general headings in the trees
LEVODOPA             ╱
   D2.92.311.242.48        D14.307.678
   D12.125.72.573.400.500  D16.538.251.575
   75; was see DOPA 1972-74
   X L-DOPA
```

```
            CENTRAL NERVOUS SYSTEM DEPRESSANTS

ANTIPARKINSON AGENTS   D14.307
   Amantadine          D14.307.106       D2.219.75.
                                         D20.388.123
   D 145*              D14.307.106.251   D2.219.75.
   Benserazide*        D14.307.140       D2.442.175
   Benztropine*        D14.307.223       D3.132.889
   Carbidopa           D14.307.232       D2.92.311.
   Dexetimide*         D14.307.250       D3.383.621.
   Diethazine*         D14.307.268       D3.494.741.
   Ethopropazine*      D14.307.499       D3.494.741.
   Levodopa            D14.307.678       D2.92.31.
   Nomifensine*        D14.307.694       D3.438.531.
```

terms from the *MeSH* Trees. In a search, telling the computer to "explode Antiparkinson Agents" will retrieve all of the articles in the database on the general term and all of the specific drugs listed underneath. Computers can definitely make information searching easier! This takes care of one concept in our search and we will probably retrieve many articles on the various drugs used to treat Parkinson Disease. But we are still left with our second concept, elderly. In *Index Medicus, you* would have to look through the drug article titles to find some indication that certain articles discussed the use of the drug in the elderly. On the computer you can add the second term, AGED, to your computer search and retrieve only those articles that are indexed under one or more of the AN-TIPARKINSON AGENTS and AGED.

The steps in developing an information search strategy that have been discussed here are summarized in Table 1-8. A flow chart indicating how to use *MeSH*, in particular, is shown in Figure 1-7. A printout from a MEDLINE search based on our sample search problem with the addition of a third concept, CLINICAL TRIALS, can be found in Table 1-9.

Table 1-8. Steps In Developing an Information Search Strategy

STEPS IN DEVELOPING AN INFORMATION SEARCH STRATEGY

1. Identify the concepts.

2. Evaluate the importance of each concept to the search results.

3. Select MeSH terms to represent each concept.

4. Conduct the search using the appropriate index or computer database.

Understanding Logical Relationships

In the database search example in Table 1-9, the computer was used to combine groups of *MeSH* search terms using logical connectors based on our initial search strategy. Computer search strategies require clear thinking about both the search terms that represent the concepts and the logical relationships among these groups of terms. Taking another look at our sample search will illustrate how the computer made these logical relationships explicit.

For THE FIRST CONCEPT, the instruction to the computer to "explode ANTIPARKINSON AGENTS" resulted in the computer linking together all of the different drug terms with the logical connector word *or*. By *"or"*ing the terms, the computer created a set in which each article retrieved contained at least one of the drug names. In the search, this set was then combined with the term AGED using the logical connector word *"and."* The result was a set in which each article retrieval contained at least one of the drug names as well as AGED. In online searching, the terms *or* and *and* take on a particular meaning. A third logical connector, *not*, which excludes a concept from the search retrieval, is also available. The logical connectors and the way in which they operate in a search is shown in Figure 1-8. The concept map previously shown in Figure 1-6 shows the way in which the connector words are used to combine terms listed under the separate concepts.

This chapter has introduced the process of information searching by explaining search strategy development using the building blocks ap-

Figure 1-7. How to Use Medical Subject Headings (MeSH)

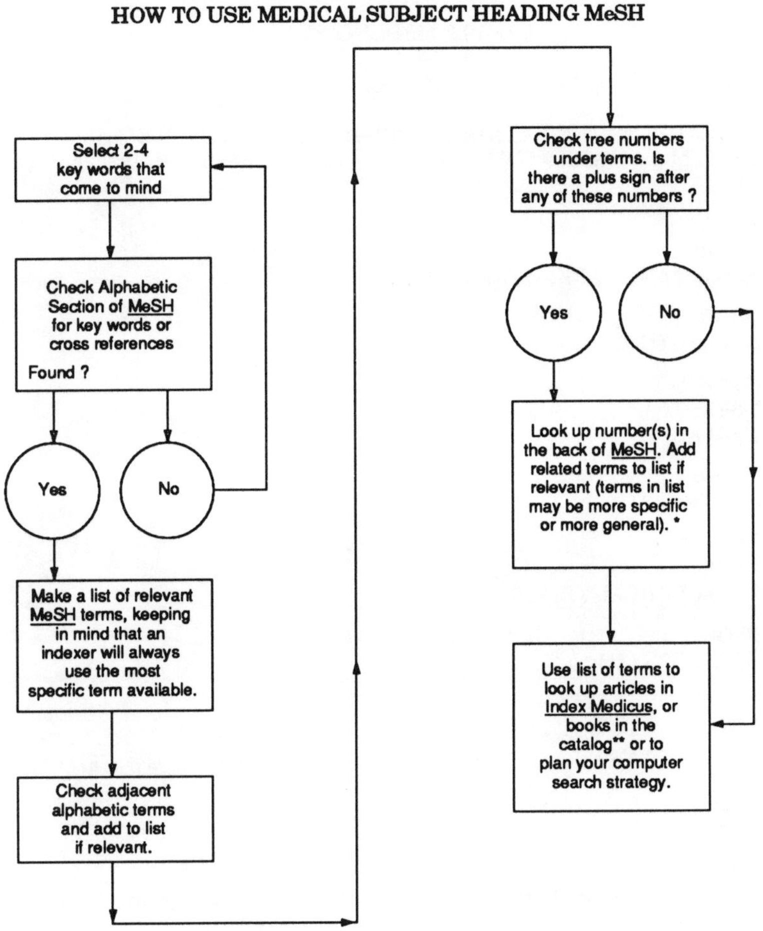

HOW TO USE MEDICAL SUBJECT HEADING MeSH

Select 2-4 key words that come to mind

Check Alphabetic Section of MeSH for key words or cross references
Found ?

Yes   No

Make a list of relevant MeSH terms, keeping in mind that an indexer will always use the most specific term available.

Check adjacent alphabetic terms and add to list if relevant.

Check tree numbers under terms. Is there a plus sign after any of these numbers ?

Yes   No

Look up number(s) in the back of MeSH. Add related terms to list if relevant (terms in list may be more specific or more general). *

Use list of terms to look up articles in Index Medicus, or books in the catalog** or to plan your computer search strategy.

*In the Tree Structures section of *MeSH,* any term with an asterisk will not be found as a heading in *Index Medicus.* These terms are considered minor descriptors and are only searchable on the computer. In order to find information on these subjects, look for the term under which this heading is indented.

**Only if your library uses the MeSH subject headings.

proach. Once the conceptual building blocks of a question are identified, search strategies for both printed indexes and computer databases can be developed using *MeSH* terms. This *MeSH* terminology can be used to search library catalogs that use NLM classification and indexes and databases in the MEDLARS family. There are other important informa-

Table 1-9. Sample MEDLINE Search

SAMPLE MEDLINE SEARCH

NLM TIME 14:39:58 DATE 90:305 LINE 675 GM#050010A

WELCOME TO THE NATIONAL LIBRARY OF MEDICINE'S ELHILL
SYSTEM. YOU ARE NOW CONNECTED TO THE MEDLINE (1988-90)
FILE.

SS 1 /C?
USER:
explode *ANTIPARKINSON AGENTS

PROG:
SS (1) PSTG (671)

SS 2 /C?
USER:
1 and AGED

PROG:
SS (2) PSTG (184)

SS 3 /C?
USER:
2 and CLINICAL TRIALS

PROG:
SS (3) PSTG (31)

SS 4 /C?
USER:
print compressed

PROG:

1
AU – Selby G
TI – The addition of bromocriptine to long-term dopa therapy in
        Parkinson's disease.
SO – Clin Exp Neurol 1989;26:129-39.

2
AU – Ceballos-Baumann AO; von Kummer R; Eckert W; Weicker H
TI – Controlled-release levodopa/benserazide (Madopar HBS): clinical
        observations and levopoda and dopamine plasma concentrations in
        fluctuating parkinsonian patients.
SO – J Neurol 1990 Feb;237(1):24-8.

3
AU – De Michele G; Mengano A; Filla A; Trombetta L; Campanella G
TI – A double-blind, cross-over trial with madopar HBS in patients with
        Parkinson's Disease.
SO – Acta Neurol (Napoli) 1989 Dec; 11 (6):408-14.

tion tools in the health sciences, in addition to those discussed, that use different kinds of subject terms and indexing approaches. Many of these other sources are discussed in detail in Chapter 2 of this book. Nevertheless, this chapter has provided you with a general knowledge of the building blocks strategy and the importance of using an authorized list of subject terms that will assist you in understanding and using many different information tools in the future.

Figure 1-8. Logical Connectors Used in Database Searching

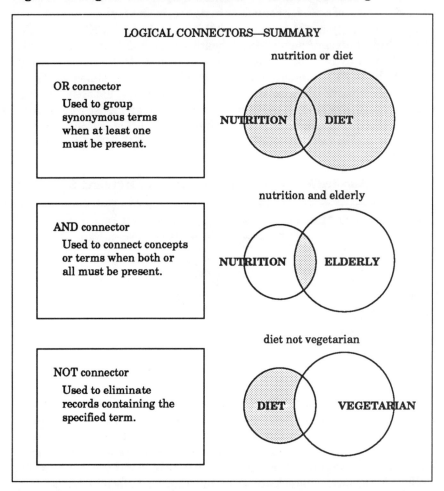

Critical Appraisal Search Strategies

When requesting a database search or conducting a search yourself, it may be useful to include a concept that relates to critical appraisal. The process of critically appraising or evaluating research literature is described in detail in Chapter 3. Database searching offers some assistance in identifying literature that meets certain critical appraisal criteria.[32] The *MeSH* terms that identify this literature are discussed here, as well as certain features of database access that make use of the computer essential for critical appraisal searching. You may want to read this discussion now, or perhaps return to it later, after gaining a better understanding of critical appraisal principles by reading Chapter 3.

In most cases, *MeSH is* used to obtain a list of terms that reflect the subject content of a search topic. For instance, in the earlier example, we were looking for journal articles on ANTIPARKINSON AGENTS and the AGED. But there are some *MeSH* headings that are used to identify particular study methods, study types or research techniques. A list of some of the more commonly used terms from *MeSH is* shown in Table 1-10. One or more of these terms can be added to a database search strategy to narrow or limit retrieval to those articles that use a particular study method. For example, the search example in Table 1-9 added the term Clinical Trials to the subject search on ANTIPARKINSON AGENTS and AGED.

Table 1-10. Selected Methods Terms Available for MEDLINE Searching

SELECTED METHODOLOGICAL TERMS AVAILABLE FOR MEDLINE SEARCHING	
Epidemiologic Methods	Drug Evaluation
Cross Sectional Studies	Drug Screening
Longitudinal Studies	Placebos
Follow-up Studies	Comparative Study
Prospective Studies	Research
Retrospective Studies	Feasibility Studies
Population Surveillance	Pilot Projects
Sampling Studies	Research Design
Evaluation Studies	Double-Blind Method
Clinical Trials	Random Allocation

In MEDLINE there are different levels of indexing available in the print and electronic products. Being aware of this is important since it affects your ability to find articles that meet critical appraisal criteria. Because of the size limitations of the printed *Index Medicus,* no more than three or four *MeSH* subject terms can be assigned to an article. Since space is less of a problem in the electronic environment, indexers have the luxury of adding extra terms. These additional terms are not usually the main point of the article, but they help to describe its content. The greater depth indexing is accessible only when using the computer. Research methods used in a study are rarely the main point of an article. For example, there may be articles under the heading CLINICAL TRIALS in *Index Medicus,* but these will be articles that specifically discuss clinical trials as a research method. In other words, the main point of the article would have to be clinical trials in order for us to find an article under that term in the printed index. In critical appraisal searching, we want to find studies that have *used* the clinical trial as a data gathering method. Retrieval at this level is available through database searching but not through the printed *Index Medicus.* The same principles of main point indexing apply to all of the bibliographic databases in MEDLARS such as Health Planning and Administration and Bioethicsline. An illustration of the greater retrieval on the computer for some of the methods terms is shown in Table 1-11.

The term CLINICAL TRIALS is a special kind of *MeSH* term known as a **check tag** in MEDLARS. This means that the term actually appears on the indexing form, and that the indexer checks the term if the article being indexed is a clinical trial. This check tag was introduced in 1980 and is defined as, "preplanned controlled studies on humans selected according to predetermined criteria of eligibility and observed for predefined evidence."[33] CLINICAL TRIALS does not assume double-blind or triple-blind studies, but the term DOUBLEBLIND METHOD can be added to the search. From 1965 to 1979 there was a check tag called CLINICAL RESEARCH that had a more simple definition, namely controlled clinical research on human beings (in contrast to uncontrolled studies on human beings or on human matter examined in vitro). If a database search covers the years prior to 1980 using Clinical Trials, the term CLINICAL RESEARCH will automatically be searched for the earlier years. Both CLINICAL TRIALS and CLINICAL RESEARCH apply to human studies only.

Table 1-11. Sample MEDLINE Retrieval for Selected Methods Terms

SAMPLE MEDLINE RETRIEVAL FOR SELECTED METHODS TERMS*		
TERM	MAIN POINT RETRIEVAL	FULL MEDLINE RETRIEVAL
Clinical Trials	256	3,738
Double Blind Method	2	1,820
Prospective Studies	2	3,145
Random Allocation	25	3,372
Explode Epidemiologic Methods	1,565	22,043

Main point retrieval includes those articles that discuss the research method as the mainpoint of the article.
Full MEDLINE retrieval also includes journal articles describing those studies that have used the study method.
Full MEDLINE retrieval is available only via computer.

*Based on a search of the NLM MEDLINE file (1988-1989) conducted in February 1989

Another useful check tag is COMPARATIVE STUDY. From 1965 through 1973 this term was used for the comparison of two or more drugs or chemicals, or two or more therapeutic, diagnostic, or determinative procedures. In 1974 the application was widened to include comparisons of any two or more concepts. The term PLACEBOS is also available for searching.

When searching back several years, check to see when the *MeSH* terms used in the search were introduced into the vocabulary. For instance, RANDOM ALLOCATION was added in 1978. Prior to 1978 it would be necessary to search for these words or other words with similar meaning in the title or abstract of the article. Keep in mind that *MeSH is* being revised and updated each year. The methods terms are scattered around in the alphabetic *MeSH* vocabulary, but groups of terms are brought together under more general terms in the *Tree Structures*. A summary of the methods terms in their tree structure configuration is shown in Table 1-12. As discussed previously, it is possible to explode categories of the *MeSH* terms so that all of the terms are collected together into one search set. All or any of these methods terms could potentially be added to a subject search to assist in identifying the research literature.

If a search result that meets all of the critical appraisal criteria is required, the following terms can be added to your content search:

1. CLINICAL TRIALS;
2. RANDOM ALLOCATION; and
3. DOUBLE-BLIND METHOD

If the searcher is satisfied with any one of these terms being present, enter CLINICAL TRIALS or RANDOM ALLOCATION or DOUBLEBLIND METHOD. If a less rigorous approach is sufficient, enter explode EPIDEMIOLOGIC METHODS or explode EVALUATION STUDIES, or explode RESEARCH, or COMPARATIVE STUDY, or PLACEBOS. Each of the preceding search statements represents a level of critical appraisal search strategy that can be combined with other subject search concepts.

Citation Indexes

Another extremely useful information tool in the health sciences, citation indexing, is based upon a completely different approach to analyzing journal literature from those discussed so far. It is worthwhile becoming acquainted with the principle behind citation indexing before reading about the specific tools in Chapter 2. The value of citation indexing is based upon the cumulative nature of scientific research. For example, if an occupational therapist wrote an article on the use of

Table 1-12. Methods Terms in Tree Structure Format

METHODS TERMS IN TREE STRUCTURE FORMAT

Evaluation Studies   E3.337
  Clinical Trials
    Multicenter Studies
    Randomized controlled trials
  Drug Evaluation
  Drug Screening
    Drug Screening Assays, Antitumor
    Subrenal Capsule Assay
    Tumor Stem Cell Assay
  Product Surveillance, Postmarketing
  Program Evaluation
  Reproducibility of Results

Research   H1.770.644
  Animal Testing Alternatives
  Clinical Protocols
  Feasibility Studies
  Human Genome Project
  Pilot Projects
  Reproducibility of Results
  Research Design
    Double-Blind Method
    Meta-Analysis
    Random Allocation*

Study Characteristics (Non-MeSH)   E5.318.760
  Analytic Studies (Epidemiology) (Non-MeSH)
    Case-Control Studies
      Retrospective Studies
    Cohort Studies
      Longitudinal Studies
        Follow-up Studies
        Prospective Studies
    Cross-Sectional Studies
      HIV Seroprevalence
  Clinical Protocols
  Clinical Trials
    Multicenter Studies
    Randomized Controlled Trials
  Feasibility Studies
  Intervention Studies
  Pilot Projects
  Sampling Studies

Study Design (Non-MeSH)   E5.318.780.300
  Double-Blind Method
  Meta-Analysis
  Random Allocation
  Reproducibility of Results
  Sensitivity and Specificity (Epidemiology)
    Predictive Value of Tests
    ROC Curve
  Seroepidemiologic Methods
  Single-Blind Method

quality circles for improving case management, he or she is likely to cite important earlier work on the subject. This article may, in turn, be cited by future authors as they continue to add to our knowledge of the subject. Citation indexes take advantage of the linking together of related works provided by the citing practices of authors.

How are citation indexes used? Let's say that we know of a great article written several years ago on evaluating the effectiveness of continuous subcutaneous insulin infusion pumps. We feel certain other pertinent studies have been done since that time and it is likely they have cited this important earlier work. So instead of selecting a subject term to start our search, we pick this article. The citation indexes, *Science Citation Index* and *Social Science Citation Index*, tell us who has cited a particular article since it was written.

This process leads to some interesting findings that differ somewhat from the results of a traditional subject approach. Using the citation indexes is particularly useful when it is difficult to identify an appropriate subject term in *MeSH* or the other indexes. Citation indexes can also be used to look at the impact of a researcher's work on others. One author has referred to citations as the "paper trails of scholarship."[34] The citation indexes are available as printed indexes and as databases. In addition to the printed citation index section that has been described, there is an author section and a permuterm section. The latter section acts as an index to the words in the title of the articles.

Current Awareness

In addition to searching for information related to problems encountered on a daily basis, most health professionals also want to develop some specific mechanisms for maintaining a general level of current awareness in their field. Joining one or more professional associations that have an annual conference and publications, such as a newsletter and journal provides an excellent base for your current awareness program, but there are also several ways in which using the library can help. Many health sciences libraries keep their current issues of journals in a special area before they are shelved with the earlier issues; this section can be checked on a regular basis. A similar arrangement may apply to new books that are received. Some libraries will send photocopies of tables of contents of specific journal titles or alert individual health professionals to new articles of potential interest.

The idea of circulating tables of contents is such a popular one that there is a commercial product based on it. *Current Contents,* mentioned earlier in this chapter as the most up to date of the indexing tools, reproduces the title pages of many journals. Indexes to keywords in the title are included as well as author addresses that are useful for requesting reprints. *Current Contents is* published in several different subject sections, including Health Services Administration, Clinical Medicine, Social Sciences and Life Sciences. This service is also available as an online database. Another service called *Reference Update* provides a weekly floppy disk full of recent citations. The latter product is compatible with the company's *Reference Manager,* a personal database management program for the microcomputer. Another electronic option for current awareness is to make use of the online databases that we discussed earlier. Most of the online search services offer a current awareness service in the form of a search based on the material added to a database in the last month. The National Library of Medicine MEDLARS system has a separate database called **SDILINE**, which stands for Selective Dissemination of Information online. A predefined search strategy can be run against this file on a monthly basis and a printout of the journal article citations can be obtained, with or without abstracts. Libraries can set up these SDI profiles to run automatically for a reasonable cost. A librarian can advise health professionals about the monthly update services that are available from the different vendors and provide the specific cost.

Information Etiquette

When information is located, it may simply be used to make a decision or to add to our own background knowledge of a subject. In at least some cases however, students and practitioners use the information contained in publications to help them write papers. Certain ethical and legal rules must be observed when using another author's work. As stated in a standard manual of writing style, in academic writing everything taken from an outside source requires acknowledgement.[35] This includes not only specific quotations and paraphrases but also information and ideas. As a general rule, the origin of anyone else's content which appears in your writing, that readers might otherwise assume to be your own, should be indicated. Failure to acknowledge the use of another person's ideas or written expressions is known as plagiarism. Authors are generally delighted to have someone else use their work, but they want to have their original work cited. Reprinting significant portions of another person's work in a publication most often requires written permission from the author and publisher of the original work.

Plagiarism
Achtert and Gibaldi point out that plagiarism is a moral offense rather than a legal one, but that it is a serious breach of the writer's responsi-

bility to acknowledge sources.[35] In academic settings, where writing and ideas are the major basis for evaluating an individual's contributions, plagiarism can have serious consequences. Academic writing includes both professional writing for publication and student papers. Plagiarism can range from quoting another person's words directly without indicating the source to simply claiming a particular argument or approach as your own without acknowledgement. As unpublished works have copyright protection in most countries, these guidelines apply equally to the use of published and unpublished materials. Plagiarism can sometimes happen quite by accident, particularly after reading a number of different sources in preparation for writing a paper, so it is wise to take precautions to reduce this possibility. For example, when taking notes from sources, be sure to record the source and complete citation. If in doubt about whether to cite a source, the best choice is usually to provide the citation.

Bibliographic Style

An author is responsible for citing sources in a standard format. The term "bibliographic style" refers to the way in which a source is cited in the text of a paper, as well as the format used in the list of references or bibliography at the end of the paper. The use of a standard bibliographic format ensures that citations will be presented in a manner that makes it easy for the reader to locate the original sources. Since readers depend upon the accuracy and completeness of citations to locate the related works, and tools such as the citation indexes input these citations into their databases, references are important. There are a number of standard bibliographic formats found in the health sciences literature, such as the "Vancouver style" used by many of the major biomedical journals.[36] Another commonly used style in the health and social sciences is described fully in the *Publication Manual of the American Psychological Association*.[37] In the case of student papers, the instructor or the school may have specified a particular bibliographic style to be used. If the paper is to be submitted for publication to a journal, the "Instructions to Authors" section published in the journal will likely indicate the style to be used. Copies of the standard bibliographic style manuals are usually kept in libraries.

Copyright

Copyright is another matter of information etiquette that deserves attention. Unlike plagiarism, which is usually considered more of an ethical breach, copyright is a legal matter. According to the copyright laws of various countries, authors' published and unpublished works are legally protected against unauthorized reproduction. In the United States the period of copyright is the life of the author plus 50 years.

A key principle used in current copyright legislation is that of "fair use." This applies not only to the use of portions of an original document in a new work but also to the photocopying of existing works. A discussion of the fair use provision, according to U.S. copyright law, is provided by Achtert and Gibaldi.[35] Many libraries provide brochures with copyright guidelines and most carry a number of standard handbooks for writers that discuss both plagiarism and copyright issues. Generally, copyright law allows for single copying for individual scholastic use, as well as single copying for teachers and limited multiple copies for classroom use. The latter arrangement is subject to a set of conditions that should be investigated more carefully if multiple copying is anticipated.

As usual, it seems that technology is racing ahead of our social and legal ability to cope with the capabilities offered by the machines. The proliferation of photocopiers has made it easier than ever before for us to reproduce previous work. In one way, this has made the lives of students and researchers much easier. Many of us find it extremely valuable to have copies of relevant publications beside us as we review evidence and prepare papers. But the photocopying boom has also created a crisis in the library and publishing world. Publishers claim that photocopying practices are cutting down on the number of original works sold. Thus, the costs of buying the original books and journals continues to increase. Another related problem involves the unauthorized copying of computer software. Many copyright laws are being revised to accommodate this new medium as a published product.

As users of research knowledge and potential authors ourselves, the legal and ethical uses of information and information resources will continue to be a matter of concern. Careful observation of information etiquette is the major means through which we can guarantee the fair use of our own scholastic and professional contributions in the future. To a large extent, we are responsible for setting standards of professional conduct in this area.

In the end, the quality of a health professional's information seeking habits depends on the individual's level of commitment to maintaining and enhancing his or her professional knowledge base. The general understanding of the information search process presented in this chapter serves as a sound basis for gaining a greater knowledge of the specific information search tools discussed in Chapter 2, and the critical appraisal criteria elaborated in Chapter 3.

References

1. Maizell RE: Continuing education in technical information services. J Chem Documentation 7:115, 1967.

2. Voigt MJ: Scientists' Approaches to Information. Chicago: American Library Association, 1961. (Association of College and Research Libraries Monograph Number 24).

3. Marshall JG, Neufeld VR: A randomized trial of librarian educational participation in clinical settings. J Med Educ 56:409-416, 1981.

4. Northup D, et al.: Characteristics of clinical information seeking: Investigation using critical incident technique. J Med Educ 58(1):873-881, 1983.

5. Farmer J, Guillaumin B: Information needs of clinicians: Observations from a CML program. Bull Med Libr Assoc 67(1):53-54, 1979.

6. Dykes MH: Beating the knowledge and technology explosion. JAMA 246:1924-1925, 1981.

7. Fineberg HV, Gabel RA, Sosman MB: Acquisition and application of new medical knowledge by anesthesiology. Anesthesiology 48:430-436, 1978.

8. Huth EJ: The underused medical literature [editorial]. Ann Intern Med 110(2):99-100, 1989.

9. Menzel H: Interpersonal and unplanned communication: Indispensable or obsolete? In Roberts EB, et al.: Biomedical Innovation. Cambridge, Massachusetts: MIT Press, 1981, p. 153-163.

10. Coleman JS, Katz E, Monzol H: Medical Innovation: A Diffusion Study. Indianapolis, Indiana: Bobbs-Merrill, 1966.

11. Friedlander J: Clinician search for information. J Amer Soc Info Sci 24:65-69, 1973.

12. Rubenstein AH, et al.: Search vs experiment: The role of the research librarian. Coll Res Libr 34:280-286, 1973.

13. Herman CM, Rodowskas Jr. CA: Communicating drug information to physicians. J Med Educ 51:189-196, 1976.

14. Thomas L: Hubris in science? Science 30:1459-1462, 1978.

15. Crane D: Invisible Colleges: Diffusion of Knowledge in Scientific Communities. Chicago, Illinois: University of Chicago Press, 1972.

16. Shibutani T: Improvised News: A Sociological Study of Rumor. Indianapolis, Indiana: Bobbs-Merrill, 1966.

17. Greene NM: Gossip and the acquisition of knowledge. Anesth Analg 57:519-520, 1978.

18. Parboosingh J, et al.: How physicians make changes in their clinical practice: A study of physicians' perceptions of factors that facilitate this process. Ann Roy Coll Phys Surg Can 19(4):429-435, 1986.

19. Currie BF: Continuing education from medical periodicals. J Med Educ 51:420, 1976.

20. Curry L, Putnam RW: Continuing education in Maritime Canada: The methods physicians use, would prefer and find most effective. Can Med Assoc J 124:563-566, 1981.

21. Stinson ER, Mueller DA: Survey of health professionals information habits and needs: Conducted through personal interviews. JAMA 243(2):140-143, 1980.

22. McCarthy S: Personal Filing Systems: Creating Information Retrieval Systems on Microcomputers. Chicago, Illinois: Medical Library Association, 1988.

23. Haynes RB, et al.: How to keep up with the medical literature: VI. How to store and retrieve articles worth keeping. Ann Intern Med 105:978-984, 1986.

24. Stibic V: Personal Documentation for Professionals: Means and Methods. Amsterdam: North-Holland, 1980.

25. Davies NE, DeVierno AA: Reimbursement for computer-assisted literature searches for patient care [letter]. New Eng J Med 319(15):1021, 1988.

26. Day RA. How to Write and Publish a Scientific Paper 2nd edition. Philadelphia, Pennsylvania: ISI Press, 1983.

27. Directory of Online Databases, Volume 9, Number 1, Jan 1988. New York, New York: Cuadra/Elsevier, 1988.

28. Haynes RB, et al.: Computer searching of the medical literature: An evaluation of MEDLINE searching systems. Ann Intern Med 103:812-816, 1985.

29. Marshall JG: How to choose the online medical database that's right for you. Can Med Assoc J 134:634-640, 1986.

30. Marshall JG: Characteristics of early adopters of end-user online searching in the health professions. Bull Med Libr Assoc 77(1):48-55, 1989.

31. Harter SP: Online Information Retrieval: Concepts, Principles and Techniques. Orlando, Florida: Academic Press, 1986.

32. Marshall JG: Sizzling search strategies: How to put some methods terms in your MEDLINE searches. Bibliotheca Medica Canadiana 5(3):88-90, 1983.

33. Charen T: MEDLARS indexing manual: Part II. Bethesda, Maryland: National Library of Medicine, 1981.

34. McCain KW: The paper trails of scholarship: Mapping the literature of genetics. Libr Quart 56:258-271, 1986.

35. Achtert WS, Gibaldi J: The MLA Style Manual. New York, New York: Modern Language Association of America, 1985.

36. International Committee of Medical Journal Editors: Uniform requirements for manuscripts submitted to biomedical journals. Ann Intern Med 108:258-265, 1988.

37. American Psychological Association. Publication Manual of the American Psychological Association 3rd edition. Washington, DC: American Psychological Association, 1983.

2

The Resources: Putting Them To Work

Linking Information Searching Resources to Practice

Lynda M. Baker

Learning Objectives
After completing this chapter, the reader will be able to:

- Compare the subject coverage of the indexes, and choose the ones that will provide the most relevant information on the topic;
- Identify the elements of a citation;
- Decide whether to access information through an index or via the computer; and
- Judge the effectiveness of a resource for a specific information need.

Introduction

In 1597, Francis Bacon stated that knowledge is power. One hundred and seventy-eight years later, Samuel Johnson elaborated on this theme: "Knowledge is of two kinds. We know a subject ourselves, or we know where we can find information upon it." The latter part of Johnson's statement is especially pertinent today with the tremendous increase in health care literature. Finding information in a health sciences library is not as difficult as it may seem. Libraries organize information in a general way. They also house resources which organize material more specifically. Knowing that particular resources exist to help in the search for information is half the battle; knowing how to use these tools is the other half.

This chapter of the book will introduce you to the indexes most widely used by health care professionals. Each resource tool will be discussed in full in order that you, the searcher, will be able to approach an index with an understanding of how the material is organized and thus, how information can be found. The computerized access to each index is included. If your library does not subscribe to a particular index in the print format, you can gain access to the information via the computer.

Most indexes are produced by organizations, for example, the National Library of Medicine (NLM), the American Psychological Association (APA), or the Kennedy Institute of Bioethics. These organizations include in their indexes those journals that cover material relevant to their emphasis. Many journals do not have a common theme throughout an issue, therefore it is common to find the same journal covered by different indexes. An example of this is *Nursing Research,* which is indexed in *International Nursing Index, Cumulative Index to Nursing and Allied Health Literature, Index Medicus* and *Science Citation Index.* Perhaps you are thinking that this duplication of journal coverage presents more problems in the search for information. Actually the converse is true: the broader the coverage, the more likely you are to find the article.

How do you decide where to start looking for information on a topic? Which index will provide the best coverage of a topic? This chapter lists the subjects covered by each index so that you can decide which one should be accessed first. But what if your institution does not subscribe to the best source? Are there alternatives? The answer is yes, because of the duplication in coverage of the journals by the different indexes.

Another question arises. When is it best to do a computer search instead of a manual one? Here are a few examples of when a computer search would be the most expedient way to find information:

1. When two or more concepts need to be discussed in the same article. EXAMPLE: the therapeutic use of streptokinase or tissue

plasminogen activator (t-PA) in myocardial infarction;

2. When you are looking for clinical or random allocation studies. Unless these words appear in the title of an article, you will miss a lot of literature by doing a manual search;
3. When the concept is brand new, it is easier to locate material via the computer. Literature is added to the computer databases faster than it is indexed in the printed indexes;
4. When you need comprehensive coverage of a topic, it is wise to do a computer and a manual search;
5. When more that one database needs to be searched to pull out all the information on a topic;
6. When you want information quickly, since it takes time to sift through indexes and write down the citations; and
7. When you only want what has been indexed in the current year.

Below are situations when a search is not worth doing:

1. When you are looking for literature on a single topic. EXAMPLE: surgical repair of femoral neck fractures. This information can be found in indexes such as *Index Medicus* under the subject heading **FEMORAL NECK FRACTURES**, with **SURGERY** as a subheading; and
2. When you do not have your topic well defined or defined narrowly enough.

Computer access to literature is fast, and can be economical if you have a well defined topic. However, computer searching should not be the only route in your search for information, as you can find many good and relevant articles by searching manually through indexes.

To help you decide whether to do a manual search or a computer search, four problems have been constructed to assist you in identifying which index to consult first, what could be an alternative and whether or not a computer search would aid in your quest for information.

PROBLEM A:

You are a physical therapist or occupational therapist working with a patient newly diagnosed as having Guillain-Barre (GB) syndrome and the patient is receiving plasmapheresis treatments. You feel your knowledge of GB is scanty. You would like general articles on this syndrome, as well as specific ones on the use of plasmapheresis and on the rehabilitation of these patients.

During your orientation to the hospital library, you remember the librarian mentioning the value of a good review article, since it provides an overview of a topic or a "synthesis of the state of knowledge in a given field."[1]

This problem requires two different approaches to the searching process, as you need both medical and rehabilitation literature.

I. Medical:

You want a review article on Guillain-Barre, as well as a few articles on the therapeutic use of plasmapheresis. Who would be writing articles on these topics, if not physicians? Therefore, start with the medical indexes: *Index Medicus, Excerpta Medica.* Section 8. *Neurology and Neurosurgery* or *Science Citation Index.*

Index Medicus has a section entitled, "Bibliography of Medical Reviews," which just lists review articles. The correct subject heading for Guillain-Barre in this index is **POLYRADICULON-EURITIS**. Start your search in this section, under this heading for a review article. You may be lucky to find an article discussing plasmapheresis in the review section but if not, turn to the general subject part of this index. Look for the subject heading **POLY-RADICULONEURITIS** and scan the column of literature listed there until you find the subheading **THERAPY**. It is in this area that you will find articles on plasmapheresis and Guillain-Barre.

In *Excerpta Medica,* key words from the article are listed in the subject index, while in the *Permuterm Subject Index* of *Science Citation Index,* words from the title are combined. In both of these indexes, you can look for either Guillain-Barre or polyradiculoneuritis, in combination with review or reviews or plasmapheresis.

II. Rehabilitation:

You can use the three indexes just discussed, or you could access the literature from an index that covers more occupational therapy and physical therapy journals.

Cumulative Index to Nursing and Allied Health Literature (CINAHL) covers many journals from the physical therapy and occupational therapy disciplines and is a good place to search for literature written by these health professionals. The subject heading is **POLYRADICULONEURITIS.**

Another index to check is *Excerpta Medica.* Section 19. *Rehabilitation and Physical Medicine.* You can look for many combinations of the terms: Guillain-Barre or polyradiculoneuritis, plus exercises, rehabilitation, activity etc. in the subject index.

You can access rehabilitation in *Index Medicus* under **POLYRADI-CULONEURITIS** by looking under the subheading **REHABILITATION**. There is some overlap among the three indexes, so you may not feel the need to check all three.

Computer Access:

A computer search is not really necessary in this case. However, one reason for choosing the computerized method is that, by looking in *Index Medicus* under the subject heading **POLYRADICULONEURITIS**, subheading **THERAPY**, you will find a lot of material on other types of therapy too. Since you are just interested in plasmapheresis, using the computer would be faster.

PROBLEM B:

As a third year nursing student, you are asked to make a presentation on the benefits of including a course on nursing ethics in the curriculum. Where should you begin to look for information to support your theory? Start your search in the nursing indexes, but think also about an index which covers educational literature and one dedicated to ethics.

I. *Cumulative Index to Nursing and Allied Health Literature.* Under the subject heading **ETHICS, NURSING,** the material is further subdivided by subheadings. In this case, look for the subheading **EDUCATION** to find information on your topic. You may have to look through a few years of the index to find some literature. Do not forget the monthly issues for the current year!

II. *International Nursing Index.* This index also covers this topic under the subject heading of **ETHICS, NURSING.** Unlike *CINAHL,* there is no subdivision of this heading, so you have to scan all the articles to find the ones most relevant to your topic.

III. *Bibliography of Bioethics.* This index is dedicated to literature on ethics, as the name suggests. The subject heading is **NURSING ETHICS/EDUCATION.** Here you may find information from books, journals or reports of organizations.

IV. *Current Index to Journals in Education.* This educational index could provide information on your topic since you are concerned with adding a course to the curriculum. Look under the heading **ETHICS.**

Computer Access:

A computer search may be of some value, although not essential since this topic is covered under a single heading in the health related indexes. However, a search of the educational database, ERIC, should be considered since **ETHICS** is a broad concept and it is best to combine **ETHICS** with other terms such as nursing, nurses, nursing education, etc. to retrieve relevant literature.

PROBLEM C:

You are an intern on the cardiac ward. During rounds, you are asked to prepare a talk on the use of anticoagulants in patients with cardiomyopathy. Since this is a medical problem, you should look in the following medical indexes for information:

   i. *Index Medicus*

   ii. *Excerpta Medica.* Section 6. *Internal Medicine*
     Excerpta Medica. Section 18.
     Cardiovascular Diseases and
     Cardiovascular Surgery

   iii. *Science Citation Index*

Computer Access:

Since there are different anticoagulant drugs and different cardiomyopathies, you would have to look under many subject headings to find information. This topic is perfect for a computer search. In some databases such as MEDLINE, searching for anticoagulant drugs is easy because all the anticoagulant drug terms can be searched by "exploding" that category. The same holds true for the cardiomyopathies. By "AND"ing these two concepts, you would retrieve articles on anticoagulants and cardiomyopathies. What would have taken hours to search manually, the computer can produce in a very few minutes.

PROBLEM D:

You are a social worker with a multidisciplinary health care team. Mr. X is ready for discharge, but the physician is hesitant to send him home, as he believes Mr. X has been subjected to some abuse by his family. You are asked to look into different treatment modalities for the family and the patient. Elder abuse is a problem that is studied by many disciplines, each having a different emphasis. Therefore, consider the perceptive from which you wish to approach the topic. Then consult a medical, psychological, allied health, or sociological index because all will present a slightly different slant of information.

I. *Index Medicus*. **ELDER ABUSE** became a subject heading in 1984. Since this index does include social work journals, it would be a good place to start your search. It will also provide medical information.

II. *Cumulative Index to Nursing and Allied Health Literature*. The correct subject heading in this index is **ABUSE OF THE ELDERLY**. This index also picks up social work journals, so the material is easy to find. Nursing literature can add another perspective to this topic.

III. *Psychological Abstracts*. The subject heading **ELDER ABUSE** was added to this index in 1988. Prior to this time, you would have had to look under **FAMILY VIOLENCE**. When a concept such as elder abuse gets added to an index under its own heading, this indicates that there is enough literature on the topic to warrant a specific heading.

IV. *Social Science Citation Index* or *Sociological Abstracts*. These two indexes should be added to your search for information, as they index a number of social work journals.

Computer Access:

This is a case where looking manually through the indexes is a wise move before doing a computer search, because there is a subject heading. However, if your library does not subscribe to these indexes, all are available on-line. A search on **ELDER ABUSE** by itself might be too broad, and you would have to think of specifics with which to narrow the retrieval, such as therapy, psychotherapy or family counseling, to name a few.

Now is the time to introduce each of the indexes alluded to in the problems. The best method for learning how to use an index is to read the information on it in this section and then use the index to find literature on a particular topic. Or, you can read the information on two different indexes and compare them, i.e. the layout of the index, the access points, the literature you find. Becoming proficient in using an index takes time and repeated effort. Do not get frustrated! If you do not succeed on your own, ask the librarian for help.

As mentioned in the previous chapter, many of the indexes are now available on compact disc. The library user can perform his/her own computer searches, usually free of charge. If this option of finding information is open to you, take advantage of it. It is a fairly easy way to find literature on your topic. But, one still needs to know the basics of each index to determine which system to access.

Index Medicus

PUBLISHER: National Library of Medicine, Bethesda, Maryland 20894.

HISTORY: This index has a long and interesting history. The first volume was published in 1879 by Dr. John Shaw Billings. Since then, it has gone through a series of slightly different names and publishers. For a more detailed picture of this fascinating story, the reader is directed to Blake's book in the bibliography of this chapter. *Index Medicus*, as it is known today, has been published by the National Library of Medicine since 1960.

COVERAGE: *Index Medicus* is one of the main indexes for biomedical literature; it indexes journal articles in medicine, nursing, occupational therapy, physical therapy, biology, nutrition, social work, chemistry, physiology, etc.

FREQUENCY OF PUBLICATION: Monthly. At the end of the year, the twelve monthly volumes are cumulated into a fourteen volume series entitled *Cumulated Index Medicus.*

ARRANGEMENT OF INDEX: The monthly issues are arranged in three sections:

1. Bibliography of Medical Reviews: This section contains the review articles indexed for that month. These articles are also indexed in the general subject section and are identifiable because the number of references at the end of the article are included with the bibliographic record;

2. Subject Section: All the articles indexed for that month are arranged under the subject headings, as they are in *Cumulated Index Medicus*. (See below for more explanation); and

3. Author Section: The citations are arranged alphabetically by first author, with "see" references from co-authors to the first author.

Cumulated Index Medicus is formatted differently. The first six volumes provide author access to the literature, while volumes 7 through 14 are dedicated to subject access. Bibliography of Medical Reviews is found in Volume 2.

1. Subject Section: The citations are indexed under major subject headings according to specificity. This means that general articles

on a topic are listed first, followed by articles under subheadings that are relevant to the topic. Subheadings also help to organize the literature. To find articles on drug therapy of a disease, look under the disease heading, scan down to the section entitled **DRUG THERAPY**, and there you will find articles of interest. This saves time because you do not have to read through pages of citations to find articles on drug therapy. Within this arrangement, the citations are organized according to the journal title, not author's name. English language articles appear before foreign ones. The layout of a citation (Figure 2-1) is as follows.

2. Author Section: The arrangement is alphabetical. The full bibliographic citation accompanies the primary author entry only. Coauthors have "see" references to the primary author.

Figure 2-1. Example of a citation from the subject index of *Index Medicus*

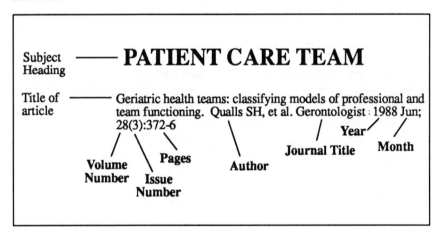

NOTES: There are several tools which are essential to use along with this index. The most important is *Medical Subject Headings,* usually referred to as *MeSH.* This thesaurus is the controlled vocabulary used by the National Library of Medicine for indexing journal articles. Changes to this vocabulary are made on a yearly basis, i.e. subject headings are added or deleted, reflecting the trends of the literature. *MeSH* lists the subject headings alphabetically in the first section, then hierarchically by categories and subcategories in the second. In the Alphabetic List section, each heading is combined with at least one alphanumeric code called Tree Structures and the year the term was entered into *Index Medicus.* There are also "see" "see under" or "see related" references. The "see" reference leads you from a nonacceptable heading to the correct one. The "see under" indicates that if you are looking for material on **GESTURES**, you have to look under the subject heading **KINESICS**. The "see related" note indicates that additional headings might bring forth more literature on your topic. For example, looking for articles on epidural injections, there is a "see related" note suggesting that you also look under the headings **ANESTHESIA, CONDUCTION** or **ANESTHESIA, EPIDURAL.**

The thesaurus also includes a list of the subheadings with notes to which categories of terms they can be assigned and a scope note on the usage of the term in this index.

The hierarchical section, Tree Structures, lists subject headings by major categories, subdividing these into more specific categories. Since it is the policy of the National Library of Medicine to index as specifically as possible, the Tree Structures can help you to narrow in on the most specific term. The converse is also true. In the Alphabetic List section, the searcher can identify which terms are broad by the inclusion of a plus (+) sign after the Tree Structure number. The following flow chart (Figure 2-2) will help the searcher work through the process of finding terms, using both sections of *MeSH.*

The second valuable tool to consult is the *List of Journals Indexed* in *Index Medicus.* This contains a list of all the short and long forms of the journal titles found in *Index Medicus.* Two sections in the back of *List of Journals Indexed* arrange the journal titles by subject and by geography.

COMPUTER ACCESS: The on-line version of *Index Medicus* is MEDLINE, which is actually a composite of three indexes: *Index Medicus, International Nursing Index* and *Index to Dental Literature.* This file is available through:

    I. National Library of Medicine, MEDLARS: MEDLINE — 1966 to the present;

    II. Dialog: MELINE Files 152, 153, 154, 155—1966 to the present; and

    III. BRS/Search Service, BRS/Colleague, BRS/After DARK, BRS/Instructor: MEDLINE (MeSH) and Backfiles—1966 to the present.

There are four separate resource tools to be used when searching the database: *Medical Subject Headings—Annotated Alphabetic List* and *Medical Subject Headings—Tree Structures.* Both of these are essential for preparing a good search strategy (Figures 2-3 and 2-4). The annotated *MeSH* provides the searcher with more notes about a subject heading, i.e. the year the term was entered into the system and what term or terms to search before the entry date. Although minor descriptors are not in the printed index, they are searchable on the computer. There is a good introductory section to the annotated version, including the new subject

Figure 2-2. Flow chart for Medical Subject Headings

HOW TO USE MEDICAL SUBJECT HEADINGS MeSH

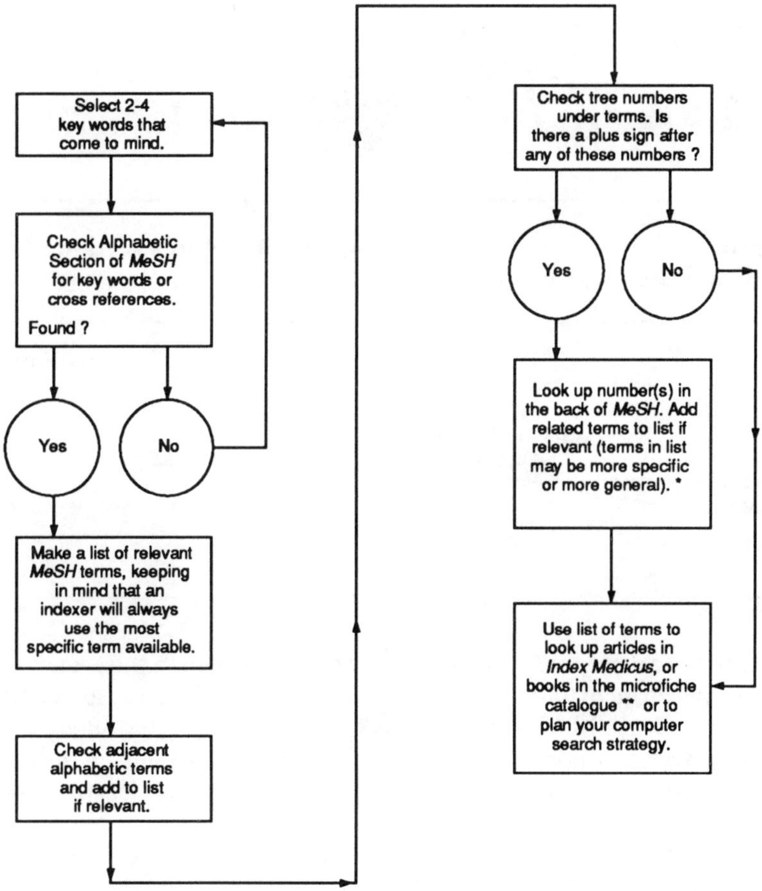

Select 2-4 key words that come to mind.

Check Alphabetic Section of *MeSH* for key words or cross references. Found ?

Yes   No

Make a list of relevant *MeSH* terms, keeping in mind that an indexer will always use the most specific term available.

Check adjacent alphabetic terms and add to list if relevant.

Check tree numbers under terms. Is there a plus sign after any of these numbers ?

Yes   No

Look up number(s) in the back of *MeSH*. Add related terms to list if relevant (terms in list may be more specific or more general). *

Use list of terms to look up articles in *Index Medicus*, or books in the microfiche catalogue ** or to plan your computer search strategy.

* In the Tree Structures section of *MeSH*, any term with an asterisk will not be found as a heading in *Index Medicus*. These terms are considered minor descriptors and are only searchable on the computer. In order to find information on these subjects, look for the term under which this heading is indented.

** Only if your library uses the NLM classificaton system.

headings and where the material was indexed previously. Two other resources that can be quite helpful are the *Permuted Medical Subject Headings* and the *List of Serials Indexed for On-line Users*, which gives the abbreviated and the long form of the journal titles. MEDLINE is also available on compact disc.

Figure 2-3. Example of an entry in Alphabetic List of Medical Subject Headings

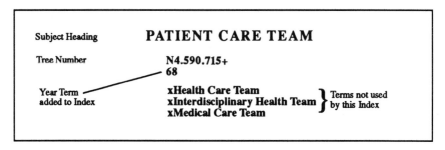

Figure 2-4. Example of an entry from Tree Structures section of Medical Subject Headings

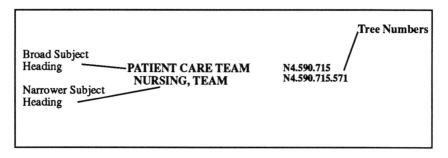

There are a number of user friendly programs which the searcher can use to perform his/her own searches from the office or home. NLM's version is Grateful Med; BRS has BRS/After Dark, BRS/Colleague, and BRS/Instructor; Dialog's MEDLINE is mounted on Knowledge Index; and Paperchase, which is produced by Beth Israel Hospital, Boston, Massachusetts.

LEARNING AIDS: A slide/tape presentation entitled "Index Medicus—an introduction and self-instructional guide" was prepared in 1980 by S.A. Bader and J.A. Schulman, George Washington University Medical Center and the Paul Himmelbarb Health Sciences Library, Washington, D.C. A recent book can help you learn to use *Index Medicus:* Strickland-Hodge, B. *How to use Index Medicus and Excerpta Medica.* Brookfield, Vermont: Gower Publishing, 1986.

For learning how to search MEDLINE via the menu driven systems or directly, two good books are available:

The Basics of Searching MEDLINE: A Guide for the Health Professional. Bethesda, Maryland: National Library of Medicine, 1989.

Feinglos, S.J. *MEDLINE: A basic guide to searching.* Chicago, Illinois: Medical Library Association, 1985.

Abridged Index Medicus

PUBLISHER: National Library of Medicine, Bethesda, Maryland 20894.

HISTORY: This smaller version of *Index Medicus* was first published by the National Library of Medicine in 1970.

COVERAGE: One hundred eighteen English journals are indexed in this index, providing the searcher with literature from core journals in different disciplines.

FREQUENCY OF PUBLICATION: Monthly.

ARRANGEMENT OF INDEX: Same as *Index Medicus*.

NOTES: Many hospital libraries subscribe to this version, while most university libraries carry all the journals covered by this index.

COMPUTER ACCESS: MEDLINE file as described above.

National Library of Medicine Published Searches

The National Library of Medicine's Literature Search Series started in 1966. Computer searches on various topics were run by the staff at NLM and made available to the public. In 1987 this series ended and three different titles became available:

1. Current Bibliographies in Medicine: Each issue covers a specific topic of interest. Different files of the MEDLARS system are searched for the citations;
2. AIDS Bibliography: This Bibliography is issued quarterly; and
3. Specialized Bibliography Series: A specific topic is chosen for each issue. The citations found in this series are from many different databases, eg. BIOSIS, EMBASE, etc. as well as the NLM databases.

Individual issues or complete sets are available from:
Superintendent of Documents
U.S. Government Printing Office
Washington, D.C. 20402.

Figure 2-5. Cumulative Index to Nursing and Allied Health Literature How to Use CINAHL

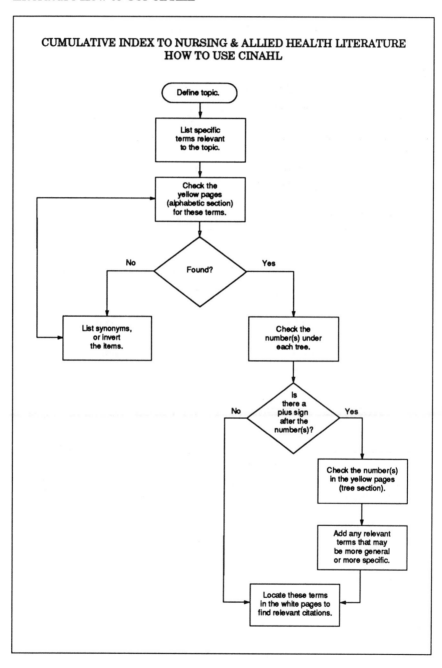

Cumulative Index to Nursing and Allied Health Literature

PUBLISHER: Cumulative Index to Nursing & Allied Health, Glendale, California 91206.

HISTORY: The first volume of *Cumulative Index to Nursing Literature* appeared in 1956, indexing articles from twelve nursing journals. Selective articles from a few health related non-nursing journals were also included. In 1967 National League for Nursing Publications was added. State nursing journals received coverage from 1972 onwards. Coverage of the literature of the American Nurses' Association started in 1968 and ran to 1970, then after a short hiatus, was reinstated in 1976.

In 1977, reflecting the new trend in health care, i.e. the multidisciplinary approach, this index changed its name to *Cumulative Index to Nursing and Allied Health Literature,* known popularly as *CINAHL,* or the red books.

COVERAGE: *CINAHL* indexes approximately 300 English language journals. Primary literature of the following disciplines is covered: nursing, occupational therapy, physical therapy and rehabilitation, laboratory technologists, medical records, social services in health care, respiratory therapy, radiotherapy and cardiopulmonary technology, emergency services, health education, surgical technology, medical and physician's assistants. In 1983 *CINAHL* added health sciences librarianship literature to the growing list of journals indexed. In addition to the 300 journals of these disciplines, *CINAHL* scans the 2600 biomedical journals from *Index Medicus* and some popular journals for relevant material. Publications of organizations such as the United States Government and the World Health Organization are included when appropriate.

FREQUENCY OF PUBLICATION: This index is published bimonthly for ten months of the year: January/February, March/April, May/June, July/August and September/October. The months of November and December are included in the cumulated volume which appears in February of the following year.

ARRANGEMENT OF INDEX: There is a subject and an author section to this index.

1. Subject Section: Since knowledge of how the information in this section is organized pivots on an understanding of CINAHL SUBJECT HEADINGS: a short discussion of the Alphabetical List and Tree Structures is necessary. The CINAHL SUBJECT HEADINGS are similar in structure to NLM's *Medical Subject Headings,* described in the section on *Index Medicus.*

Figure 2-6. Entry from Alphabetical List section of *CINAHL*

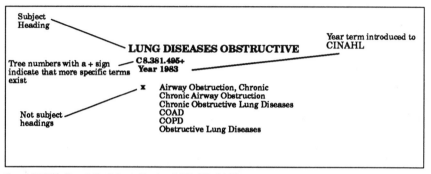

Figure 2-7. Entry from Tree Structure section of *CINAHL*

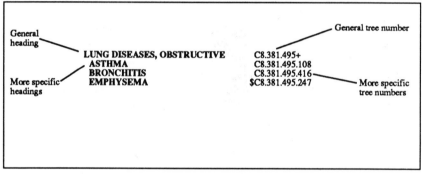

Found in the yellow pages of the annual issue or the January/
February issue, CINAHL SUBJECT HEADINGS is divided into two parts:

A. The Alphabetical List

B. The Tree Structures.

The Alphabetical List contains all the subject headings or key terms
under which the literature is indexed. Each term is assigned at least one
Tree Structures number. The dollar sign ($) beside some of the alphanu-
meric codes indicates that the terms to which it is assigned are different
from NLM's Medical Subject Headings. The only time this information
is important is if you are planning to use the same search terms in *Index
Medicus.* The terms with the dollar signs beside the numbers are
probably not in *Index Medicus,* or there is some variation in the entry.[2]

The Tree Structures section reflects another way of organizing the
subject headings, this time by categories and subcategories. Within the

Figure 2-8. Entry from the Subject section of *CINAHL*

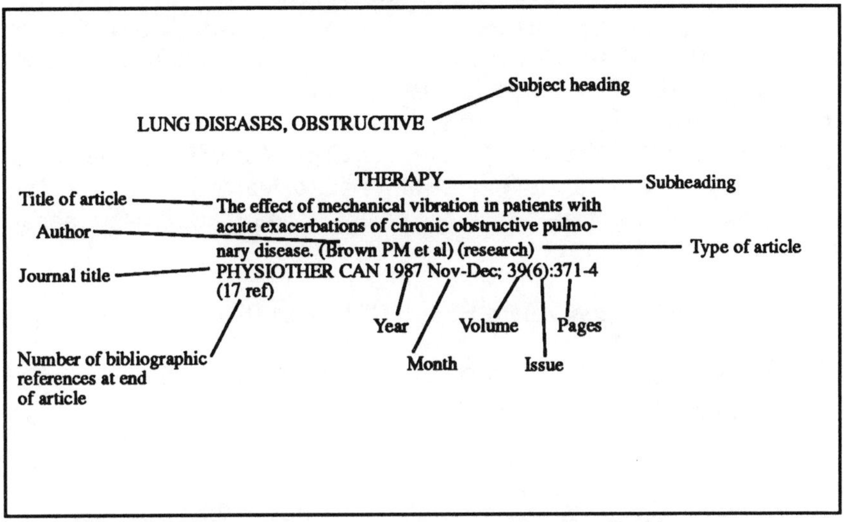

Copyright 1988, *Cumulative Index to Nursing & Allied Health Literature*, Glendale
Adventist Medical Center, Glendale, California. Reprinted with permission.

categories, the subject terms are arranged in hierarchical order, from the
broadest concept to the narrowest. Using both the Alphabetical List and
the Tree Structures allows the user to choose the most specific subject
headings relevant to his/her information needs. The following chart will
help the user through this process.

The Subject Section (white pages) of *CINAHL* contains the bibliographic citations, indexed under the CINAHL SUBJECT HEADINGS.
Subheadings, such as diagnosis, etiology, therapy, etc., can be added to
some of the subject headings. An article that specifically discusses the
therapy of an illness is indexed under the subheading THERAPY and not
under the general heading. Figure 2-8 is an example of a citation from
the Subject Section.

2. Author Section: The citations are arranged alphabetically under
   the name of the first author. Co-authors are listed as "see" references that refer the searcher to the primary author.
3. Journal and Serials Indexed Section: This section contains the
   short and long forms of all the journal titles indexed.

The addresses for the journals can be found in the annual cumulated
edition.

NOTES: *CINAHL* adds descriptor notes to some of the citations,
indicating the type of article: research; research, nursing; pictorial;

exam questions and case study, etc. These descriptors are helpful in determining whether an article is relevant to the needs of the searcher.

Twenty-eight book publishers submit books to *CINAHL.* These books are listed in the appendix "New Nursing and Allied Health Books" under CINAHL SUBJECT HEADINGS. This provides an easy method for keeping up to date with books in your area of interest.

COMPUTER ACCESS: In 1983 *Cumulatilve Index to Nursing & Allied Health Literature* became available on-line. Abstracts from some of the nursing journals have been included on-line since 1986. This database is accessible through:

I. Dialog: Nursing & Allied Health (CINAHL) File 218—1983 to the present.
II. BRS/Search Service, BRS/Colleague, BRS/After Dark and BRS/Instructor: Nursing & Allied Health Database (NAHL)—1983 to the present.

Nursing & Allied Health is available on compact disc.

LEARNING AIDS: *CINAHL* has produced a slide/tape presentation entitled "Diane Discovers the Red Books" which gives step by step instructions on how to use *Cumulative Index to Nursing and Allied Health Literature.*

International Nursing Index

PUBLISHER: The American Journal of Nursing Company, New York, NY 10019-2961.

HISTORY: *The International Nursing Index* (INI) began in 1966. It was, and still is, published by the American Journal of Nursing Company in cooperation with the National Library of Medicine, using the computer facilities of NLM's MEDLARS (Medical Literature and Retrieval System).

COVERAGE: *INI* provides worldwide coverage of nursing literature. Two hundred seventy nursing journals are indexed, as well as relevant nursing articles from the 2600 biomedical and allied health journals from *Index Medicus,* the National Library of Medicine's bibliographies and NLM's Health and Administration database (Healthline).

FREQUENCY OF PUBLICATION: This nursing index is published quarterly. The first three volumes are soft covered; the final volume, hardbound, is the annual cumulated volume.

ARRANGEMENT OF INDEX: *International Nursing Index is* divided into two sections: subject and author. The subject headings used are from NLM's *MeSH (Medical Subject Headings)* and from the Nursing Thesaurus which is found only in the annual cumulation. The latter acts as

Figure 2-9. Example of entry from *International Nursing Index*

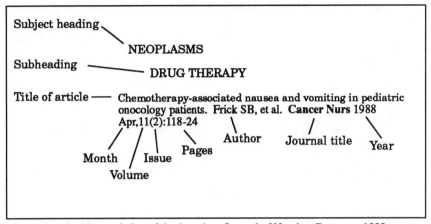

Reproduced with permission of the American Journal of Nursing Company, 1988.

a supplement to *MeSH*. It guides the user to the proper *MeSH* heading using "see" references. The "see also" and "see related" references indicate other terms under which relevant literature might be found. The Thesaurus is updated annually.

1. Subject Section: Articles are listed alphabetically by journal title under the *MeSH* subject headings. The citation includes the title of the article, the author's name, the short form of the journal title in bold type, followed by the year, the month, the volume and issue numbers and the pages. Foreign articles are distinctive by the square brackets enclosing the title. The language is abbreviated to three letters and appears to the right of the citation. Since the short form of the journal title is used throughout the index, the searcher must turn to the "Journals Indexed" section to find the complete title. An example from the Subject Section is found in Figure 2-9.

2. Author/Name Section: The citations are arranged alphabetically by author. The entry is under the first author's name only; the coauthors have "see" references by their names directing the user to the initial author. Anonymous literature is listed alphabetically under the journal name at the end of the Author/Name Section.

3. NURSING CITATION INDEX: The addition of this important section to *INI* occurred in 1986. The *Nursing Citation Index* is produced by the Institute for Scientific Information and provides another access route to the literature. The references in the bibliography of

Figure 2-10. Example of entry from *Nursing Citation Index*

Author of
cited article   Title of Journal

HUGULEY CM   Volume

Year

81 CANCER 47 989   Page

Cited   HAUGHEY BP   ONC NURS F   15   315   88
article   LAUVER D   CANCER NURS   11   51   88

Citing authors; these   Volume Page   Year
authors have cited
Huguley's 1981 ariticle   Title of Journals
from CANCER, Volume 47,
page 989 in their articles

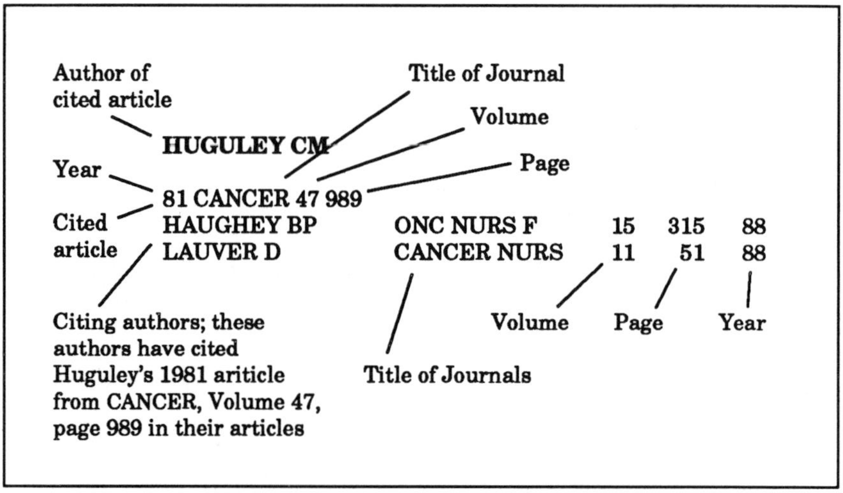

Reproduced with permission of the American Journal of Nursing Company and the Institute for Scientific Information

an article are a valuable source of information. They often lead the user to more articles on the topic. However, they refer to work done in the past. The *Nursing Citation Index* does the opposite. It indicates who has cited a particular article since it was published, thus leading the searcher forward in time. In the following example, the author CM Huguley wrote an article in the journal *Cancer* in 1981, Volume 47, page 989. In 1988 the two authors listed below this entry quoted this particular article of Huguley's in their articles. The two authors, BP Haughey and D Lauver, are referred to as "citing" authors since they cited in their bibliographies a reference to Huguley's work.

4. Five other sections are worth noting, four of which can aid in the process of keeping you up to date with nursing publications. One is "Publications of Organizations and Agencies, 19—to 19—" which lists current publications by country, subdivided by organization. Another section, "Nursing Books Published 19—to 19—" introduces books written by or for nurses within the current year. The books are listed by country, then by broad subject areas as required. The third section, entitled "Dissertations for 19—to 19—," provides a list of doctoral dissertations by nurses arranged alphabetically by institution. The fourth section "Nursing Related Data Sources, 19—," is a compilation of studies and/or surveys relating to nursing

resources. *INI* also provides the searcher with the MEDLARS/ MEDLINE centers throughout the world.

COMPUTER ACCESS: *International Nursing Index* is one of the three indexes making up the National Library of Medicine's MEDLINE file; the other two are *Index Medicus* and *Index to Dental Literature*. See the section on *Index Medicus* for database information.

LEARNING AIDS: There is no specific learning guide to *INI*. However, one might apply the same principles discussed in "Index Medicus: An Introduction and Self-Instructional Guide" to learn how to use *International Nursing Index*.

Excerpta Medica

PUBLISHER: Excerpta Medica, subsidiary of Elsevier Science Publishing, Amsterdam, The Netherlands.

HISTORY: *Excerpta Medica* was first published in 1946.

COVERAGE: Biomedical literature, both research and clinical, is covered on a world-wide basis by this European indexing and abstracting resource. There are fifty-two sections to this index, each having its own editor, including: *Rehabilitation and Physical Medicine* (Section 19); *Gerontology and Geriatrics.* (Section 20); *Pharmacology* (Section 30); *Psychiatry* (Section 32); *Occupational Health and Industrial Medicine* (Section 35); to name a few.

FREQUENCY OF PUBLICATION: The number of issues for each section varies from eight to ten per year.

ARRANGEMENT OF INDEX: There is a table of contents, depicting the general topics either alone or further subdivided under which the literature is indexed.

1. Abstract Section: The citations are listed by abstract number under the general topic headings or the subdivisions. The title of the article is in bold print, followed by the author's name, the organization to which the first author is affiliated, the title of the journal in italics, the year, the volume/issue and the pages in brackets. Each citation has an English abstract, even if the original article is not in English.
2. Subject Index: This section allows the searcher to focus on the specifics. Key words selected from the articles are printed in bold typeface followed by other terms relevant to the article. This permits the searcher to decide quickly if the citation is on the topic. The abstract number follows this string of words.
3. Author Index: The author's last name, initials and abstract number are given. In the last issue of the year, there is a cumulative Subject

Index and Author Index.

NOTES: There are two useful tools to help the searcher use *Excerpta Medica. The Guide to the Classification and Indexing System* has a listing of all the sections, the table of contents for each, as well as the audience to whom each of the 52 sections is oriented. The chapter entitled "Guide to Subject Index Terminology" displays the terms found in the sections. The numbers following the terms indicate in which sections material on this topic can be found; the most relevant section is in bold type. The other publication is *List of Journals Abstracted,* alphabetically displaying the journal titles indexed by this service.

COMPUTER ACCESS: The literature is covered from 1974 to the present on the following databases:

I. Dialog: EMBASE Excerpta Medica. File 72,172,173
II. BRS/Search Service, BRS/Colleague, BRS/Instructor: EMBASE (EMED) Backfile and Merged File (EMEZ).
EMBASE is available on compact disc.

LEARNING AIDS: Strickland-Hodge, B: *How to Use Index Medicus & Excerpta Medica.* Brookfield, Vermont: Gower Publishing, 1986.

ERIC
(Educational Resources Information Center)

In 1964, ERIC was part of the U.S. Office of Education but, in 1972, came under the National Institute of Education. Information on education was gathered by 16 clearinghouses throughout the United States and published in an index called Research in Education. Each clearinghouse (See Table 2-1) focused on a specific aspect of education; the same holds true today. However, the producers of ERIC realized that the journal literature was not being covered adequately and, in 1975, made some changes to reflect the growth of this body of literature. Today there are two printed sources for educational material. *RIE Resources in Education* covers documents, while *Current Index to Journals in Education (CIJE)* indexes journal articles. These will be discussed separately.

RIE Resources in Education

PUBLISHER: Superintendent of Documents, Department of Education, Washington DC 20202

Table 2-1. ERIC Clearinghouses

ERIC Clearinghouses

CE ADULT, CAREER, AND
VOCATIONAL EDUCATION
Ohio State University
National Center for Research in Vocational
Education
1960 Kenny Road
Columbus, Ohio 43210-1090
(614) 486-3655; (800) 8484815

CG COUNSELING AND PERSONAL SERVICES
University of Michigan
School of Education, Room 2108
Ann Arbor, Michigan 48109-1259
(313) 764-9492

CS READING AND COMMUNICATION SKILLS
Indiana University
2805 East 10th St., Smith Research Ctr
Bloomington, Indiana 47405-2373
(812) 335-5847

EA EDUCATIONAL MANAGEMENT
University of Oregon
1787 Agate Street
Eugene, Oregon 97403-5207
(503) 686-5043

EC HANDICAPPED AND GIFTED CHILDREN
Council for Exceptional Children
1920 Association Drive
Reston, Virginia 22091-1589
(703) 620-3660

FL LANGUAGES AND LINGUISTICS
Center forApplied Linguistics
1118 22nd St, N. W.
Washington, DC 20037-0037
(202) 429-9551

HE HIGHER EDUCATION
George Washington University
One Dupont Circle, N.W, Suite 630
Washington,DC 20036-1183
(202) 296-2597

IR INFORMATION RESOURCES
Syracuse University
School of Education
Huntington Hall, Room 030
Syracuse, New York 13244-2340
(315) 423-3640

JC JUNIOR COLLEGES
University of California at Los Angeles
Mathematical Science Building, Room 8118
Los Angeles, California 90024-1564
(213) 825-3931

PS ELEMENTARY AND EARLY
CHILDHOOD EDUCATION
University of Illinois
College of Education
805 West Pennsylvania Avenue
Urbana, Illinois 61801-4897
(217) 333-1386

RC RURAL EDUCATION AND SMALL, SCHOOLS
Appalachia Educational Laboratory
1031 Quarier Street, PO. Box 1348
Charleston, W.V. 25325
(304) 347-0400

SE SCIENCE MATHEMATICS, AND
ENVIRONMENTAL EDUCATION
Ohio State University
1200 Chambers Road, Room 310
Columbus, Ohio 43212-1792
(614) 292-6717

SO SOCIAL STUDIES/SOCIAL SCIENCE
EDUCATION
Indiana University
Social Studies Development Center
2805 East 10-m St.
Bloomington, Indiana 47405-2373
(812) 335-3838

SP TEACHER EDUCATION
American Association of Colleges for
Teacher Education
One Dupont Circle, N.W, Suite 610
Washington, DC 20036-2412
(202) 293-2450

TM TESTS, MEASUREMENT, AND EVALUATION
American Institutes for Research (AIR)
3333 K Street NW
Washington, DC 20007
(202) 342-5000

UD URBAN EDUCATION
Teachers College, Columbia University
Box 40
525 West 120th Street
New York, New York 10027-9998
(212) 678-3433

Used by permission. The Oryx Press, 2214 N. Central Ave., Phoenix, AZ 85004. Copyright ©
1988 ERIC Clearinghouses

HISTORY: *RIE Resources in Education* began in 1975 with Volume 10.

COVERAGE: Documents and reports pertaining to education are collected by the 16 clearinghouses. The material is indexed and abstracted for inclusion in *RIE*.

FREQUENCY OF PUBLICATION: Monthly with semi-annual cumulative indexes.

ARRANGEMENT OF INDEX: There are six sections to this index. You will want to start with the Subject Index first, then refer to the Document Resumes to get the full information on the document.

1. Subject Index: Subject terms are taken from the *Thesaurus of ERIC Descriptors* and from the Identifier Authority List used by the ERIC indexers. Under the descriptor is the title of the document and the ED number.

2. Document Resumes: Documents are arranged alphanumerically by an ED (ERIC document) number, clearinghouse prefix and clearinghouse accession number. Most often, you will be concerned with the ED number only. A lot of information is given with each citation. The most important include:
   - ED number
   - author name
   - title of document
   - organization from which the document originated
   - publication date
   - descriptive notes
   - from whom to order the document and the price
   - abstract
   - descriptors or subject headings

3. Author Index: The author's name, title of document and the ED number are included.

4. Institution Index: Material is arranged by institution, title of document and ED number.

5. Publication Type Index: In this section, the documents are listed according to type, i.e. guides, books, viewpoints, historical materials, etc. and corresponding code numbers. The title of the document and the ED number are included.

6. Clearinghouse Number/ED Number: For most casual users of *RIE*, this section would not be of much use.

NOTES: Material from this index is available in microfiche or paper copy from the following:
ERIC Document Reproduction Service (ERDS)
3900 Wheeler Avenue
Alexandria, Virginia 22304

Current Index to Journals in Education (CIJE)

PUBLISHER: Oryx Press, Phoenix, Arizona 85004.
HISTORY: This index started in 1975.

Figure 2-11. Example of entry from subject index

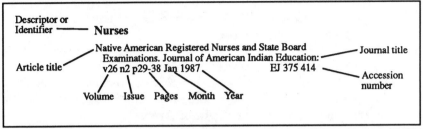

Figure 2-12. Example of a Citation from the Main Entry Section

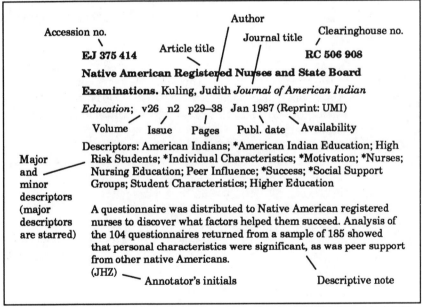

COVERAGE: Journal literature on education.

FREQUENCY OF PUBLICATION: Monthly with cumulative semi-annual indexes.

ARRANGEMENT OF INDEX: There are five sections. Start with the Subject Index to see if there is any literature relevant to your topic.

1. Subject Index: The subject headings are taken from the *Thesaurus of ERIC Descriptors* and ERIC's Identifier Authority List.

           Subject term
           Title
           Journal source, volume, issue, pages, month and year
           EJ (ERIC journal) number

2. Main Entry Section: The entries are arranged by a clearinghouse code and an EJ (ERIC journal) number.
3. Source Journal Index: This section provides the user with a list of the journals indexed, their addresses, subscription prices and where reprints of articles can be ordered.
4. Author Index: This is arranged alphabetically.
           Author's name
           Title of article
           EJ number
5. Journal Contents Index: This section provides the user with the title of the journal and a list of the articles from that journal with the EJ numbers.

NOTES: The material in this index can be obtained from the original journal. If the library does not carry the journal, users can obtain a reprint of the article from UMI Article Clearinghouse, 300 North Zeeb Road, Ann Arbor, Michigan 48106-1346 or through the interlibrary loan department of the library.

    COMPUTER ACCESS: Both *RIE* and *CIJE* compose the ERIC Datatbase.

I. Dialog: ERIC File 1—RIE—1966 to the present
    CIJE—1969 to the present
II. ORBIT Search Service: ERIC—1966 to the present
III. BRS/Search Services, BRS/Colleague, BRS/After Dark and BRS/Instructor: Educational Resource Information Center (ERIC)—1966 to the present.

ERIC is available on compact disc.

Psychological Abstracts

    PUBLISHER: American Psychological Association, Inc., Arlington, Virginia 22201.

    HISTORY: Psychological literature has been covered since 1894 with the commencement of *Psychological Index,* which continued publication until 1935. *Psychological Abstracts* began in 1927 and continues to the present.

    COVERAGE: Many journals and serial publications as well as *Dissertation Abstracts International,* are scanned regularly for articles

Figure 2-13. Entry from the Subject Index (*Psychological Abstracts*)

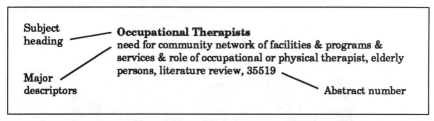

relevant to behavior and psychology.

FREQUENCY OF PUBLICATION: Monthly. The annual or cumulative index arrangement has varied over the years. At first, only one volume was needed to contain all of the information for a given year. However, a two volume set soon became necessary. Then another change took place whereby January-June material appeared in two volumes along with an index; the same was true for the July-December material. Thus, there were two sets, each with a different volume number, for the same year. In 1984 with Volume 71, the arrangement of the material changed again. The subject index is divided between two volumes; there is one author index plus four volumes housing the abstracts.

ARRANGEMENT OF INDEX: In the monthly issues, the information is indexed under one of the sixteen (16) major content classifications or a subsection of these classifications. The citations, complete with the abstract and abstract numbers, are listed alphabetically by author under these headings. In the back of each monthly issue, there is a Brief Subject Index section giving only one subject heading and the abstract numbers relevant to this heading. There is also an Author Index listing the author's name and abstract number.

The records from the twelve monthly issues are cumulated into an annual set that consists of two Subject Indexes, one Author Index and four volumes for the citations.

1. Subject Index: The subject headings under which the literature is indexed are selected from the *Thesaurus of Psychological Index Terms.* The terms assigned to the articles are deemed major or minor. The major ones reflect the main emphasis of the article and it is only these which are printed in the subject indexes; the minor headings are searchable only on the computer. Under the major subject headings are "index phrases," key words, which most accurately reflect the content of the article. An abstract number

Figure 2-14. Entry from Abstract Section (Psychological Abstracts)

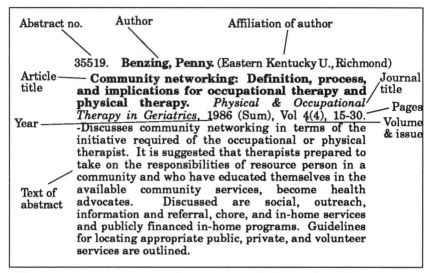

Abstract no. Author Affiliation of author

35519.   **Benzing, Penny.** (Eastern Kentucky U., Richmond)

Article title — **Community networking: Definition, process, and implications for occupational therapy and physical therapy.** *Physical & Occupational Therapy in Geriatrics,* 1986 (Sum), Vol 4(4), 15-30.

Journal title

Pages

Year — -Discusses community networking in terms of the initiative required of the occupational or physical therapist. It is suggested that therapists prepared to take on the responsibilities of resource person in a community and who have educated themselves in the available community services, become health advocates. Discussed are social, outreach, information and referral, chore, and in-home services and publicly financed in-home programs. Guidelines for locating appropriate public, private, and volunteer services are outlined.

Volume & issue

Text of abstract

accompanies these phrases. If the *Thesaurus is* not available, the Subject Index provides the user with the necessary help through the "see" reference, leading the user to the preferred term.

2. Author Index: Since 1984 the full bibliographic citation and abstract number are listed alphabetically under first author's name. A total of four authors are listed, followed by "et al." A "see" reference beside a name indicates that this person is a co-author of the article and refers the searcher to the primary author and the relevant abstract number.

3. In the volumes containing the abstracts, the citations and abstracts are arranged under each of the 16 major content classification headings or their subsections. Within these sections, the citations are alphabetical by first author. The institutional address of the first author is given. Non-English article titles are translated and inserted into square brackets; English abstracts are included. The number of references at the end of the article is noted in brackets. Figure 2-14 is an example.

NOTES: In 1988 the fifth edition of the *Thesaurus of Psychological Index Terms* was published. This tool can be used to identify the correct terms to use to find information in the indexes or via the computer. The indexing terms are accompanied by the following: the date the term was added to the *Thesaurus;* a scope note; and broader, narrower, or related terms.

COMPUTER ACCESS: *Psychological Abstracts* is available on-line on:

I. Dialog: PSYCINFO File 11—1967 to the present
II. BRS/Search Service, BRS/Colleague, BRS/After Dark, BRS/Instructor: PsycINFO (PSYC)—1967 to the present.

There is also a current awareness file, which provides brief indexing and full bibliographic information on newly published material; this material is added to the full database each month. Material from *Dissertation Abstracts International is* not included in this file. This file is searchable through:

I. Dialog: PsycALERT File 140—updated weekly
II. BRS/Search Service, BRS/Colleague, BRS/After Dark:
    PsycALERT (PSAL)—current materials only, updated weekly.

Psychological Abstracts is available on compact disc.

LEARNING AIDS: In 1980 the American Psychological Association prepared a slide/tape presentation entitled "Guide to Psychological Abstracts." It guides the searcher through the monthly and cumulative indexes.

Science Citation Index

PUBLISHER: Institute for Scientific Information, Philadelphia, PA 19104.

HISTORY: The Institute for Scientific Information started publishing *SCI* in 1961.

COVERAGE: *SCI* indexes literature from the scientific disciplines including medicine, nutrition, behavioral sciences, substance abuse, and a few nursing journals. The allied health professional should use this index in conjunction with *Social Science Citation Index (SSCI)* which is described below.

FREQUENCY OF PUBLICATION: The index is published bimonthly with an annual cumulation. There is a ten year cumulated set from 1955-1964 and several five year sets: 1965-1969, 1970-1974, 1976-1979 and 1980-1984.

ARRANGEMENT OF INDEX: There are three distinct parts to *SCI: Permuterm Subject Index, Source Index* and *Citation Index.*

Figure 2-15. Permuterm Subject Index

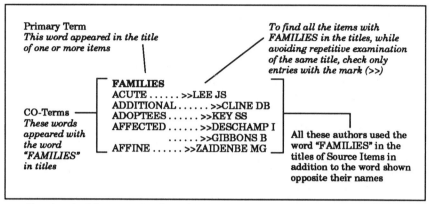

Reprinted with permission from the Science Citation Index®. Copyright by the Institute for Scientific Information®, Philadelphia, PA, USA.

1. *Permuterm Subject Index:* This is the first place to start if you wish to find information on a topic. The arrangement of this index is different from all the other indexes previously described as this index combines key words from the title of the article. A key word, exactly as it appears in the article title, is printed in large type across the top of a column. Listed underneath are words or phrases that appear in conjunction with that key word, plus the last name and initials of the author who used those words in the title of his/ her article. The searcher then goes to the *Source Index* to find the full citation which is listed under the author's name.

2. *Citation Index:* This index is based on the philosophy that authors cite in their bibliographies other papers that are relevant to their topic. Therefore, when looking for additional information on a

Figure 2-16. Entry from *Citation Index*

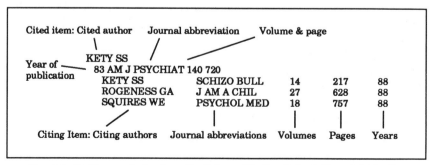

Reprinted with permission from the Science Citation Index®. Copyright by the Institute for Scientific Information®, Philadelphia, PA, USA.

particular subject, this is a valuable tool to search. However, the searcher must start with a paper on the topic. For example, you have an article written in 1983 by SS Kety. To see if anyone has quoted this paper since it was written, you would turn to *Citation Index,* starting with the 1983 edition and working forward in time. Figure 2-16, taken from the September/October 1988 issue, shows a list of this author's publications that have been cited for this time period and are arranged by year, journal title, volume number and the number of the first page. By matching the article in hand to each of these identifiers, the user will be provided with a list of authors who have cited Kety's paper in their bibliographies. The citing author's name is given along with the journal title, volume number, page and year. With this information, you can go to that journal to find the article or refer once again to the *Source Index* for the complete citation. By looking up the citing authors' articles, you now have more recent material on your topic.

3. *Source Index:* The *Source Index* is the author index. The citations are entered under the name of the first author; then the coauthors are listed, followed by the title of the article, the name of the journal, the volume and issue numbers, the pages, the year and the number of references. The address of the first author is included. The first part of the *Source Index,* called the Corporate Index, lists material by organization and geographical location.

Figure 2-17. Example of entry from *Source Index*

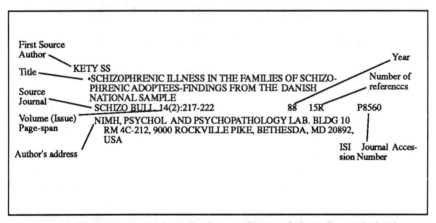

NOTES: A useful companion tool to SCI is *SCI Science Citation Index Guide and Lists of Source Publications.* The *Guide* section provides a detailed description on how to use the index, while the *Lists of Source*

Publications part lists: a) the long and short forms of journal titles, b) the address of the publisher of the journal and c) a subject and a geographical arrangement of the journals covered by SCI.

COMPUTER ACCESS: *Science Citation Index* is available on-line through:

I. DIALOG: SCISEARCH FILES 34,432,433, 434-1974 to the present.

There is also a user friendly product; Sci-Mate Software System is the menu driven system produced by ISI. There are three components to this package: The Searcher, The Manager and The Editor. The Searcher is for on-line searching. The Manager is the program for manipulating the citations, i.e. editing or sorting. The Editor is for formatting and printing your bibliography in many different styles.[3] More information on this system can be obtained by writing to:

Institute for Scientific Information
3501 Market Street
Philadelphia, PA 19104

Science Citation Index is available on compact disc.

LEARNING AIDS: The Institute for Scientific Information has many good information brochures as well as a slide/lecture presentation called *Science Citation Index (SCI)* which shows how *SCI* is organized and should be used.

Social Science Citation Index

PUBLISHER: Institute for Scientific Information, Philadelphia, PA 19104.

HISTORY: The Institute for Scientific Information started publishing *Social Science Citation Index (SSCI)* in 1969.

COVERAGE: Literature in the social sciences field is covered, including occupational therapy, physical therapy, nursing, educational research, family studies, social work, geriatrics/gerontology, health policy, library and information sciences, psychology, psychiatry, statistics and women's studies, to name a few of interest to the health science professional.

FREQUENCY OF PUBLICATION: Three times a year plus an annual cumulation.

ARRANGEMENT OF INDEX: The setup of this index is almost the same as *Science Citation Index* described above. There are three sections: *Permuterm Subject Index, Source Index,* and *Citation Index.* The major difference occurs with the information provided in the *Source Index.* The citation is the same, i.e. author, co-author(s), title of journal article, name of the journal, volume and issue numbers, pages, year, and number of references. Following this is a list of all the references from the article: author's name, year, journal title (short form), volume number and page.

COMPUTER ACCESS: *SSCI* is available through:

I. Dialog: SOCIAL SCISEARCH File 7—1972 to the present
II. BRS/Search Service, BRS/Colleague, BRS/After Dark,
    BRS/Instructor: Social SCISEARCH (SSCI)—1972 to the present.

Current Contents

PUBLISHER: Institute for Scientific Information, Philadelphia, PA 19104.

The Institute for Scientific Information (ISI) publishes *Current Contents* for eight different disciplines. The ones of interest to health professionals are: *Life Sciences, Clinical Medicine, Social & Behavioral Sciences, Arts & Humanities,* and the newest one, *Health Services Administration.*

These small publications appear weekly and contain the table of contents from the latest issues of journals. Since different subject areas are covered by the five listed above, the searcher has a wide range of journal literature to peruse. The user can order the articles he/she wants from ISI or from the author, whose address is included in the "Author Index & Address Directory" section, or can wait until the journal appears on the library shelves.

COMPUTER ACCESS: *Current Contents* is available through:

I. Dialog: Current Contents Search (File 440)—1988 to the present.
II. BRS/Search Service, BRS/Colleague, and BRS/After Dark:

1. Current Contents Search (CCON)—most current 6 months, updated weekly
2. Current Contents: Arts & Humanities (ARTS)—6 month rolling file, updated weekly
3. Current Contents: Social & Behavioral Sciences (BEHA)—6 month rolling file, updated weekly
4. Current Contents: Clinical Medicine (CLIN)—most current 6 months, updated weekly
5. Current Contents: Life Sciences (LIFE)—most current 6 months, updated weekly.

Current Contents on Diskette is a new product of ISI. It is available for IBM, IBM compatible or Macintosh microcomputers. There are two editions: J-1200 gives you exactly the same coverage as the printed *Current Contents/Life Sciences*; the J-600 edition covers 600 core journals in different disciplines. For more information on this product, you can write to:

Institute for Scientific Information
3501 Market Street
Philadelphia, PA 19104

Hospital Literature Index

PUBLISHER: American Hospital Association, Chicago, IL 60611.

HISTORY: *Hospital Literature Index (HLI)* has been published since 1945.

COVERAGE: The emphasis of this index is on health care administration and organization. Journals directly related to health care or hospital administration, health planning and health care delivery are indexed by the staff of the American Hospital Association (AHA) Resource Center. All types of health care facilities are included, such as hospices, mobile health units, multi-institutional systems, etc. Other journals are scanned for relevant articles, as are the citations from NLM's MEDLARS database. Only English language material is indexed.

FREQUENCY OF PUBLICATION: Quarterly. The last quarterly issue is incorporated into the annual cumulated volume.

ARRANGEMENT OF INDEX: There is a subject and an author section in both the monthly issues and the cumulated volume. The subject headings and the relevant subheadings have been chosen from *Medical*

Figure 2-18. Entry from Subject Section of Hospital Literature Index

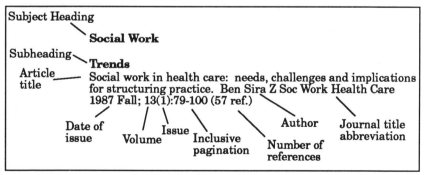

Subject Headings thesaurus produced by the National Library of Medicine. Some of the headings considered by NLM to be minor descriptors are incorporated as major headings because they are specific to literature covered by this index.

1. Subject Section: The citations are organized alphabetically by journal title. If more than one article appears from the same journal, the citations are arranged alphabetically by the first author's name. The format of the citation is identical to that found in *Index Medicus*.

2. Author Section also called the Name Section: The citations are listed alphabetically by first author. Co-authors receive a "see" reference by their names, directing the searcher to the primary author.

NOTES: There are some other helpful sections in *HLI*. The "Journals Indexed" section lists the abbreviated and the full title of the journals indexed for the particular issue. The annual volume contains the journal titles for all four quarters. Another section entitled "Recent Acquisitions" keeps the searcher abreast of new journals, books and audiovisual material acquired by the AHA Resources Center. The latter two are indexed under the same subject headings as those used in the index. New journals are listed at the end of this section under the heading "Journals."

COMPUTER ACCESS: *Hospital Literature Index* is available on three systems:

I. National Library of Medicine's MEDLARS: Healthline—1975 to the present
II. Dialog: Health Planning and Administration File 151—1975 to the present
III. BRS/Search Service, BRS/Instructor, BRS/Colleague and BRS/After Dark: Health Planning and Administration (HLTH)—1975 to the present.

Documents retrieved from this file are from three sources: the relevant journals indexed for the MEDLINE file, the journals indexed for *Hospital Literature Index* and documents cited in the Health Planning Series of the Weekly Government Abstracts. The source of each citation is added to the record, so the searcher knows from whence it came, i.e., MED from the MEDLINE file, AHA from *HLI* and NP from the Health Planning Series.

LEARNING AIDS: The American Hospital Association Resources Center has recently published a small, very informative guide entitled: "A User's Guide to the *Hospital Literature Index.*" The guide can be obtained from:
American Hospital Association Resources Center
840 North Lake Shore Drive
Chicago, Illinois 60611.

Bibliography of Bioethics

PUBLISHER: Kennedy Institute of Ethics, Washington, DC 20057.

HISTORY: Three companies have published *Bibliography of Bioethics* since 1975: Volumes 1-6 by Gale Research Company, Detroit, Michigan; Volumes 7-9 by Free Press, New York, New York; and Volume 10 onward by the Kennedy Institute of Ethics. The information has always been gathered through ongoing research at the Kennedy Institute.

COVERAGE: English language literature on ethical issues relating to health care is culled from many sources for this index, including journal articles, databases, court decisions, government documents, audiovisual material, newspapers and books.

FREQUENCY OF PUBLICATION: Annually.

ARRANGEMENT OF INDEX: The introductory section explains in detail the layout of the index which also includes the following sections: List of Journals Cited, Subject Entry Section, Bioethics Thesaurus, Title Index and Author Index. A short note on each of these follows.

Figure 2-19 Example of a government document citation

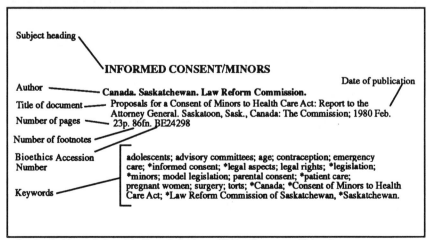

Reprinted with permission of the Kennedy Institute of Ethics, Georgetown University.

Figure 2-20. Example of a priority journal citation with abstract

Subject heading

Author

PATIENT CARE/DRUGS

Title of article

Pagination

Conrad, Peter. The noncompliant patient in search of autonomy.

Name of journal —— HastingsCenterReport. 1987Aug;17(4): 15-17.20fn.
BE24511.

Number of footnotes

Volume & Issue
Date of publication

Bioethics
Accession
Number

attitudes; central nervous system diseases; chronically ill;
*drugs; motivation; *patient care; *patients; *physician-
patient relationship; physicians; *self determination; *self-
regulation; survey; treatment refusal

Keywords

Abstract

From a medical perspective, patients who do not comply with the doctor's order
are usually seen as deviant, and deviance requires correction. But many
chronically ill people view their behavior differently, as a matter of
self-regulation. In this light noncompliance supports people's desires for
independence and autonomy, desires that align closely with the therapeutic goals
of caregivers (journal abstract).

Reprinted with permission from the Kennedy Institute of Ethics, Georgetown University.

Figure 2-21. *Bioethics Thesaurus* entry

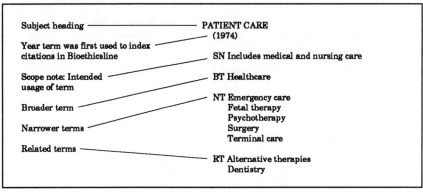

Subject heading ——————————— PATIENT CARE
(1974)

Year term was first used to index
citations in Bioethicsline

SN Includes medical and nursing care

Scope note: Intended
usage of term

BT Healthcare

NT Emergency care
Fetal therapy
Psychotherapy
Surgery
Terminal care

Broader term

Narrower terms

Related terms ————————————— RT Alternative therapies
Dentistry

Reprinted with permission from the Kennedy Institute of Ethics, Georgetown University.

1. List of Journals Cited: The journals which are indexed for that particular edition of *Bibliography of Bioethics* are listed alphabetically.
2. Subject Entry Section: The subject headings are taken from the *Bioethics Thesaurus*. The citations appear alphabetically, be they court decisions, government publications or journal articles. Full

bibliographic information for each entry is provided: the author or organization; title of article; journal title in italics; year; volume; issue,if relevant and pages. Keywords are provided; the most specific are indicated by asterisks. Abstracts are written for priority journal articles and court decisions.

3. *Bioethics Thesaurus:* The subject headings in this Thesaurus represent the controlled vocabulary used by the Kennedy Institute of Ethics to index the literature. All the headings are annotated; some have more notes than others. The information given could include: the year the term became a heading; what the heading was before the year of entry; a scope note indicating the usage of the term; related, narrower or broader terms; and a "use for" statement serving as an indicator to the acceptable term for this index.

4. Title Index/Author Index: The entries in both sections are listed alphabetically with numbers indicating the page on which the citation may be found.

COMPUTER ACCESS: *Bibliography of Bioethics* is searchable through:

I. National Library of Medicine's MEDLARS: Bioethicsline—1973 to the present.

A publication is available for new searchers: *Searching BIOETHICSLINE: A Basic Manual for the Novice Searcher*. It can be purchased for $5.00 (U.S.) from:
Bioethics Information Retrieval Project
Kennedy Institute of Ethics, Georgetown University
Washington, DC 20057

Nutrition Abstracts And Reviews

PUBLISHER: C-A-B International, Slough, SL2 3BN, U.K.
HISTORY: In 1931, under the direction of the Imperial Agricultural Bureaux Council, the Medical Research Council and the Reid Library, *Nutrition Abstracts and Reviews* was created. It was felt that nutrition literature was too scattered and the time had arrived when an index dedicated just to nutrition was needed. This index split into two sections in 1977: Series A: Human & Experimental; and Series B: Livestock Feeds and Feeding. It is now prepared by the C-A-B International Bureau of Nutrition.
COVERAGE: Journals on a world-wide basis are scanned for relevant literature on nutrition.

FREQUENCY OF PUBLICATION: Monthly.

ARRANGEMENT OF INDEX: There is a table of contents in each issue which lists five major headings: technique, foods, physiology & biology; human health & nutrition; and disease & therapeutic nutrition. Under these terms are more specific headings, e.g., lipids, leafy vegetables, minerals, diet studies, etc. Journal articles are listed under both categories of terms. Nonjournal information is entered under the headings of reports, conferences and books.

1. Abstracts: The citations are listed numerically under the broad and the more specific headings. The layout of the citations is as such: the name of the author(s), the title of the article in bold print, the name of the journal in italics, the year, the volume, the issue number and the pages. In square brackets is the language of the article abbreviated to two letters and the number of references in the bibliography. Abstracts, present for most of the articles, are in English. If the original article is not in English, a translation of the title is inserted in square brackets before the original title. The address of the first author is given.

2. Author Index: The information is straightforward, the authors' names and abstract number(s) are arranged in alphabetical sequence.

3. Subject Index: How the key terms in this section were chosen is not explained, but it appears that the main topic of the article is printed in bold face, the minor descriptors and the abstract number(s) are indented underneath.

COMPUTER ACCESS: This index has been mounted on three North American systems:

    I. Dialog: C-A-B Abstracts Files 50, 53—1972 to the present
   II. CAN/OLE: C-A-B (C-A-B Abstracts)—1972 to the present
  III. BRS/Search Service, BRS/Colleague, BRS/After Dark: C-A-B—Human Nutrition (NUTR)—1973 to the present.

References

1. Kass EH: Reviewing Reviews. In Warren KS (Ed): Coping with the Biomedical Literature: A Primer for the Scientist and the Clinician. New York, New York: Praeger, 1981, p. 79.

2. Fishel CC. CINAHL list of subject headings: A nursing thesaurus revised. Bull Med Libr Assoc 73:153-159, 1985.

3. Saari DS, Foster GA: Head-to-head evaluation of the Pro-Cite and Sci-Mate bibliographic database management systems. Database 12 (1):22-38, 1989.

Bibliography

Blake, John B., ed. Centenary of Index Medicus. Bethesda, Maryland: U.S. Department of Health and Human Services, Public Health Services, National Institute of Health, National Library of Medicine, 1980.

Chen, Ching-Chih. Health Sciences Information Sources. Cambridge: MIT Press, 1981.

Fishel, Carolyn C. "The Nursing & Allied Health (CINAHL) Data Base: A Guide to Effective Searching." Medical Reference Services Quarterly 4 (1985):1-16.

Morton, Leslie T. and Godbolt, Shane, eds. Information Sources in the Medical Sciences. 3rd ed. London: Butterworths, 1984.

On-line Databases in the Medical and Life Sciences. New York: Cuadra/ Elsevier, 1987.

Roper, Fred W. and Boorkman, Jo Anne. Introduction to Reference Sources in the Health Sciences. 2nd ed. Chicago: Medical Library Association, 1984.

3

Critical Appraisal: Analyzing the Information

Linking Research to Practice

Renee M. Williams

Learning Objectives

After completing this chapter, the reader will be able to:

- Identify what critical appraisal is;
- Describe the usefulness and importance of critical appraisal skills;
- Discuss some of the critical appraisal criteria used to evaluate the health care literature;
- Discuss the methodological criteria used to evaluate the effectiveness of therapy; and
- Apply these critical appraisal guidelines to a patient management problem.

Critical Appraisal

Critical appraisal involves the ability to be able to evaluate the validity and applicability of health care literature and to incorporate the results of this assessment into patient management.[1] How does one evaluate a study that has been published? This is what critical appraisal is all about. It is based on the professional belief that, for clinicians to be effective in the daily management of their patients, they must base their care on sound scientific evidence that they are doing more good than harm.[1] For instance, having found several articles on your topic of interest, you will need to determine whether the articles are useful to you in your clinical practice. Critical appraisal will give you the necessary skills to determine how applicable the clinical articles are. For clinicians to do more good than harm, they need to be current in their reading of the health care literature and they need to understand, evaluate and apply the evidence in the published data to their daily practice.

Why Critical Appraisal is Important

With the rapid increase in health care publications, finding and using the literature are essential skills that practitioners need to know in their day to day clinical decision making so that they can keep up to date and are better able to select patient treatments that do more good than harm. Clinicians need to be familiar with skills not only in how to retrieve health care information but also in how to critically appraise clinical articles. Learning to read an article critically and to apply its results to clinical practice is a fundamental skill that all clinicians must have.[2,3] Health care professionals need to develop and be competent in library searching and critical appraisal skills so that they can determine the quality and applicability of the material reported in clinical journals.[4,5] For practitioners to change their methods of practice clinically, they must be able to assess the evidence presented in the published journals.

Research is an ever growing source of objective information that can serve as a force for increasing professional effectiveness. Reading research articles critically and applying their findings to clinical practice are ways of linking research to practice. Because research is often reported in stilted, obscure, jargon language, clinicians need help with interpreting, applying and communicating published data. Research information that has been published must be relevant to clinicians for them to use it. Since reading clinical journals is a major source of continuing education,[6,7] clinicians need assistance to acquire and improve their self-directed learning skills[8] which are dependent on their ability to find and evaluate information.[9] Clinicians may not apply research findings from journal articles that they have read because they lack the skills necessary to understand and evaluate the articles.[10,11] A failure to use research findings may result in the best intentioned practitioners doing more harm than good to their clients. The reader who becomes familiar with the methods of assessing research will find the task of reading, understanding, evaluating and communicating the evidence documented in the clinical journal articles simplified.

Evaluating the Literature

There are numerous textbooks in the various health care professions that fully describe the "how to" of clinical research.[13-17] Critical appraisal is an integral component of the clinical research process. How do you evaluate a study? When you are evaluating a clinical study or when you are about to embark on developing a clinical trial, how have previous studies in that area of clinical interest been conducted? Are the results valid and applicable to my patients? Can I use them in my study? This is basically what critical appraisal is all about. Although the critical appraisal process is directed toward the "consumers" of research done by others rather than the "doers" of research, nevertheless, it is an essential component of research. For example, when searching for information on the effectiveness of a treatment and having located several articles on the topic of interest, how do you determine whether the articles will be useful to you in your clinical practice? Familiarity with various criteria on how to assess the literature is a necessary aspect of clinical practice that all health care professionals must have.

The Clinical Epidemiology and Biostatistics Department at McMaster University, Hamilton, Ontario, Canada has developed a series of methodological criteria upon which to evaluate the health care literature.[18] These standards are straightforward, common sense guidelines that are used to analyze and assess the literature. Critical appraisal guidelines have been developed to assess the use of a diagnostic test,[19] the clinical course and prognosis of disease,[20] the etiology or causation of health and disease,[21] the efficacy and effectiveness of a therapy,[22] the quality of clinical care[23] and the economic aspects of treatments.[24,25] These methodological criteria provide a scientific approach to determine the validity and usefulness of evidence presented in published health care literature. It is a framework for the integration of the critical appraisal of evidence to patient management decisions. Some of these guidelines are summarized in Table 3-1.

Table 3-1. Some Methodological Criteria for Critical Appraisal of Clinical Research Literature

DIAGNOSTIC TEST	PROGNOSIS
Was there an independent "blind" comparison with a "gold standard" of diagnosis?	Was an "inception cohort" assembled?
Did the patient sample include an appropriate spectrum of disease?	Was the referral pattern described?
Was the referral pattern described?	Was complete follow-up?
Was reproducibility and observer variation determined?	Were objective outcome criteria used?
Was the term "normal" sensibly defined?	Was the outcome assessment blind?
If part of a cluster of tests, was the test's overall contribution assessed?	Was adjustment for extraneous prognostic factors carried out?
Was the test described well enough to permit its exact replication?	
Was the "utility" of the test determined?	

CAUSATION	THERAPY
Is there evidence from true experiments in humans?	Was the assignment of patients to treatments really randomized?
Is the association strong?	Were all clinically relevant outcomes reported?
Is the association consistent from study to study?	Was the study recognizably similar to your own?
Is the temporal relationship correct?	Were both statistical and clinical significance considered?
Is there a dose response gradient?	
Does the association make epidemiological sense?	Is the treatment feasible in your practice?
Does the association make biological sense?	Was complete follow-up achieved?
Is the association specific?	
Is the association analogous to a previously proved causal association?	

Criteria Used to Evaluate
the Effectiveness of Therapy

Health care professionals must develop critical appraisal skills in order to evaluate the clinical and research evidence published in the literature. Since all health care professionals are involved in identifying and applying treatments that do more good than harm, the critical appraisal emphasis in this book will focus on the methodological criteria used to distinguish useful from useless or even harmful therapy.[22] For a detailed explanation of the other critical appraisal guidelines, the reader is referred to the textbook written by D.L. Sackett, R.B. Haynes and P. Tugwell.[1] Appendix A is an article entitled "How to read clinical journals: V. To distinguish useful from useless or even harmful therapy" and was published in the *Canadian Medical Association Journal* 124:1156-1162, 1981. This article will serve as a basis for the evaluation, interpretation and application of the critical appraisal skills for assessing the effectiveness of therapy. After reading this article, continue with the critical appraisal worksheet[26], which is used along with the methodological criteria for determining the effectiveness of therapy.[22]

This article was originally published in the *Canadian Medical Association Journal*, Volume 124 May 1, 1981. See the appendix for the complete article.

The Critical Appraisal Worksheet

The Critical Appraisal Worksheet[26] presented in Figure 3-1 is useful as it acts as a guide in applying the methodological criteria when assessing the health care literature. This worksheet[26] is used along with the article entitled "How to read clinical journals: To distinguish useful from useless or even harmful therapy."[22]

The reader should complete a separate Critical Appraisal Worksheet[26] for each article that is assessed. The critical appraisal evaluation should be based, if possible, on more than one journal article. Since many of the details needed to assess the credibility and applicability of the data presented are often buried in the text of the article, appraising the literature may be a time consuming process. However, you must not become discouraged. As you become more familiar with applying and utilizing these skills, you will find that, as you continue to read clinical journals, you will become more time efficient and accurate. The use of the methodological criteria[22] and the Critical Appraisal Worksheet[26] should help to simplify this task. The following is a discussion of the criteria found in the Critical Appraisal Worksheet.

Criteria in the Critical Appraisal Worksheet

The criteria outlined in the worksheet utilize the methodological guidelines of:

1. *Was the Design Architecture Appropriate?*
The design architecture refers to the type of research design, strong or weak, that was carried out in the study. This guide looks at the basic design of the study.

Figure 3-1. Worksheet for the Critical Assessment of an Article About a Preventative or Therapeutic Health Intervention

Worksheet for the Critical Assessment of an Article About a Preventive or Therepeutic Health Intervention	
Citation_____	
GUIDE	COMMENTS
1. Was the design architecture appropriate? [ ] Yes [ ] No [ ] Can't tell	1. i. (Was similarity between groups documented? Prognostic stratification) ii. Specify any biases that may be operating and the direction of their influence on the results.
2. Were all relevant health outcomes reported? [ ] Yes [ ] No [ ] Can't tell	2. (Mortality, as well as morbidity?; Deaths from all causes?; Quality of life; Are the measurement methods reproducible and valid?; Was the outcomes assessment "blind"?)
3. Were the study patients (population) recognizably similar to your own? [ ] Yes [ ] No [ ] Can't tell	3. (Eligibility criteria?; primary or tertiarty care?)
4. Were both clinical/administrative importance and statistical significance considered? [ ] Yes [ ] No [ ] Can't tell	4. (If statistically significant, was difference clinically important?; If not statistically significant, was study big enough to show an important difference if it should occur?)
5. Is the maneuvre (health intervention) feasible in your setting? [ ] Yes [ ] No [ ] Can't tell	5. (Available?; affordable?; sensible?; were contamination and co-intervention avoided?; Was it "blind"?; Was compliance measured?)
6. Were all patients who entered the study accounted for in its conclusion? [ ] Yes [ ] No [ ] Can't tell	6. (Were drop-outs, withdrawals, non-compliers, and those who crossed over handled appropriately?)
CONCLUSIONS:	

a. *Random Allocation*

The randomized clinical trial (RCT) is the strongest research design. RCTs are comparative studies in which the assignment of subjects to either the experimental or the control group is done on a purely random basis. That is, each subject has an equal chance (50%) of being assigned to either group. Random assignment attempts to eliminate any bias in the groups that may lead to erroneous outcomes or conclusions. Bias may be defined as systematic error or "difference between the true value and that actually obtained due to all causes other than sampling variability."[27] Randomization assumes that any important intervening variable, such as age, sex, severity of disease, etc., will be equally distributed between the groups.

Even with randomization, it may occur that, by chance, one group may end up with, for example, more males or older patients, thus affecting the results of the study. If there are no RCTs in the journal articles that you have located, you will have to use articles with other study designs. To determine if the study has been randomized, simply look for key terms such as "random allocation" or "random trial" in the title, abstract or the methods section of the article. Study designs have been discussed in various epidemiological and statistical textbooks.[13,14,28-30]

b. *Comparability of Study Groups and Prognostic Stratification*

Although random allocation attempts to produce comparability of the study groups, this method does not necessarily ensure that the groups will be similar with regard to all important variables. Prognostic stratification prior to randomization is a method of making the study groups comparable with regard to important prognostic factors. This involves distributing (stratifying) any factor (such as age, sex, severity of illness) that may affect the results of the trial, equally amongst the study groups in an effort to minimize its influence on the results.

2. *Were All Relevant Health Outcomes Reported?*

This guide asks if all clinically relevant patient outcomes were reported. The intent of this section is to determine how well the outcome measurements used in the article have been described. It basically looks at the methods of assessing patients and the key results.

a. *Mortality as Well as Morbidity*

Has mortality, as well as other clinically relevant morbidity results, been reported? What were the patient outcomes? How well are they described?

b. *Explicit, Objective Outcome Criteria*

The clinical outcomes should be explicit and objectively defined. Are the measurement methods used acceptable and valid (that is, are they measuring what they should be measuring)? Was the outcome assessment "blind"? If the assessments were "blind," the group allocation would be unknown to the observers. "Blindness" in a clinical trial helps to reduce potential bias.

3. *Were the Study Patients (Population) Recognizably Similar to Your Own?*

This guide asks if the patients in the study are *recognizable* and if the patients are *similar* to the patients in your practice? Were the eligibility and exclusion criteria well stated? How were the patients diagnosed? What were the patients' key sociodemographic and clinical status? Is it a primary or tertiary care setting? What is the location and level of care? It is important to know the answers to these questions so that, if these patients are similar to your own, you can apply the results to your own patients.

4. *Were Both Clinical/Administrative Importance and Statistical Significance Considered?*

This guide asks whether the results of the study were both clinically and statistically significant. If the results were statistically significant, were they clinically important?

a. *Clinical/administrative significance*

Clinical/administrative significance refers to the *importance* of a difference in clinical outcomes between treated and control patients, and it is usually described in terms of the *magnitude* of a result.[22] Clinical significance is generally based on clinical judgment, that is, it is a judgment call. For example, if the therapy in the experimental group means less hospitalization days for your patient, then you can say that the treatment is clinically significant. However, if this same therapy causes serious side effects, you will want to reconsider whether to use the treatment, even though the stay in the hospital is decreased. When determining clinical significance, you need to weigh all the pros and cons of the results before a decision can be made.

b. *Statistical significance*

Statistical significance tells us whether a difference is likely to be *real* and is a statement of the likelihood that this difference is due to chance alone.[22] For example, if the intervention in the experimental group is statistically significantly better than the control group, there is statistical significance. However, if there is an increased incidence of deaths in the experimental group, one can say that the therapy is not clinically significant.

c. *Adequacy of sample size*

Since the number of patients in a study is one of the determinants of statistical significance, are there enough patients in the study to show statistical significance? If the results are not statistically significant, was the study big enough to show an important clinical difference if it should occur? For detailed discussions on the topic of sample size estimation, the reader is referred to other references.[31-33]

5. *Is the Maneuver (Health Intervention) Feasible in Your Setting?*

This section should describe the exact intervention. Is the reader able to implement the maneuver in a similar manner to that described in the article?

a. *Replicable description of maneuver*

The maneuver should be described in sufficient detail so that the reader is able to replicate it. Who did what? To whom? When? How often? For how long? And under what circumstances? Is the intervention available in your practice? Is the maneuver affordable? Is it sensible?

b. *Contamination and co-intervention*

Contamination and co-intervention are two specific biases that should be avoided in any clinical trial. Contamination refers to the bias that occurs when the control group accidentally receives the experimental treatment; co-intervention refers to the bias that occurs when additional therapeutic and diagnostic acts are performed on the experimental but not the control group. If either of these biases occur, the clinical outcomes in both the experimental and the control groups will be affected. One way to overcome co-intervention is to make both the patients and the clinicians "blind" as to who is receiving which treatment.

c. *Patient and provider compliance*

Compliance refers to how well the patients, as well as the health care workers, followed the treatment maneuvers. An example of patient compliance is — How well have the groups followed the maneuvers or treatment regimes? An example of provider compliance is — Have the patients have been diagnosed correctly?

6. *Were All Patients Who Entered the Study Accounted For in its Conclusion?*

This guide addresses the number of subjects who entered the study and asks about the missing subjects (dropouts, withdrawals, noncompliers, crossovers, etc.) at the conclusion of the trial. Were the dropouts, withdrawals, noncompliers and crossovers handled properly? Was complete follow-up achieved?

Conclusion

It is unusual for a study to fully satisfy all six methodological standards presented above. When assessing and designing studies, clinicians should realize the relative importance of each of these methodological criteria in order to determine whether they will accept or discard the results of the trial.

Patient Management Problems

The following section will present some examples of patient management problems. These are clinical problems that are similar to those that practitioners may face in their day to day clinical practice. They deal with identifying and applying treatments that will do more good than harm.

To integrate literature searching and critical appraisal skills, some common information seeking routes and the application of critical appraisal criteria to the articles that were found will be discussed. The reader should realize that within the information searching and critical appraisal processes, if inadequate results are found, it may be necessary to restart the search.

Objectives for this Section

I. To familiarize the reader with some common information searching routes in order to find health care information that will answer the patient management problems;

II. To assess the quality of the article(s) that was located by using the critical appraisal criteria on the effectiveness of therapy and the Critical Appraisal Worksheet; and

III. To determine whether the article(s) is useful in solving the patient problem.

To accomplish the above objectives, the reader should:

1. Read the following problems carefully and choose one to pursue;
2. Explore the common manual literature searching tracks such as *Index Medicus, Cumulative Index to Nursing and Allied Health Literature (CINAHL), Science Citation Index,* etc.;
3. Use the computerized literature searching routes such as MEDLINE, Nursing and Allied Health (CINAHL), etc., (There is a cost for these searches, but it is quite reasonable);
4. Locate several articles likely to be of good quality on the patient problem that has been chosen; and
5. Assess the quality of the articles using the methodological criteria on effectiveness of therapy.[22]

Problem #1

As a member of an active rehabilitation team working with stroke inpatients, you have noticed that, despite intensive therapy, many of your patients have not regained functional use of their arms. In fact, some of them have developed a glenohumeral subluxation of their hemiplegic shoulder. You are wondering if using functional electrical stimulation (FES) would be useful. Based upon the best evidence you can find, will the FES treatments do more good than harm?

Problem #2

A newly diagnosed client with seropositive rheumatoid arthritis, whose symptoms have been present for less than a year, is under your care. Her current medical regimen consists of entrophen 650 mg TID, and Naprosyn 250 mg BID. She has had no involvement with any of the health care professionals on the rheumatology team until she was referred to you.

The rheumatology ward of your hospital has a multidisciplinary education program for people with rheumatoid arthritis. The aim of the program is to teach clients more about rheumatoid arthritis and how it is managed. You think that your client would benefit from the program; she has two young children and a husband at home and is reluctant to be admitted into the hospital. She is, however, willing to come in as an outpatient daily for the one hour sessions. She also suggests that she would probably pick up as much information by reading books and pamphlets as she would gain from attending the classes. To help you decide whether this woman should attend the educational program, you do a literature search. Having read the published evidence, what would you recommend to your client?

Problem #3

Pelvic floor exercises are an important part of prenatal and postnatal exercise programs. These exercises are recommended and taught as a means of prevention and treatment for incontinence of urine. As a nurse on the maternity ward, you notice that many of your patients, despite the fact that they have been given instructions in pelvic floor exercises, complain of urinary incontinence postpartum. You are wondering if an intensive regime of pelvic floor muscle exercises would be helpful. Based upon the best published evidence you could find, will these treatments do more good than harm?

Information Searching Routes

Table 3-2 illustrates a general information searching route that is a useful guide in obtaining literature in health care. Information can be obtained either manually or through requesting or conducting a computerized database search. Although there is a charge for computerized searching, the advantages outweigh the costs. Manual searches can be very effective; however, computerized searches require less time to do and are more efficient since the searcher is able to incorporate several subject headings and concepts together. In this way, the information can be retrieved from several sources. It is important to realize that when a manual search is done, manpower costs should be considered. Depending upon the time that the searcher wants to spend, manual searches are useful when the searcher wants to scan the literature to acquire an overview of the topic of interest.

As previously discussed in Chapter 1 of this book, since the information in journal articles is more current than the information published in general and specialty textbooks, clinical journals, rather than textbooks, will be used to find information on the patient management problems presented above. Since research terms such as **CLINICAL TRIALS, CLINICAL RESEARCH, RANDOM ALLOCATION, DOUBLE-BLIND METHOD, PLACEBO** and **COMPARATIVE STUDY** are available as *MeSH* headings, a MEDLINE (the electronic version of *Index Medicus)* search will be conducted. Also, since much of the allied health and nursing literature is found in NURSING AND ALLIED HEALTH LITERATURE (the electronic version of *Cumulative Index to Nursing and Allied Health Literature),* various computerized database searches will be done.

Table 3-2. Information Searching Routes

INFORMATION SEARCHING ROUTES

Manual Information Searching Routes
- General textbooks
- Specialty textbooks
- Reference source
- Journal articles via *INDEX MEDICUS* or *CUMULATED INDEX MEDICUS*
- Journal articles via *CUMULATIVE INDEX TO NURSING & ALLIED HEALTH LITERATURE* (CINAHL)
- Journal articles via *INTERNATIONAL NURSING INDEX* (INI)
- Journal articles via *CURRENT INDEX TO JOURNALS IN EDUCATION*
- Journal articles via *PSYCHOLOGICAL ABSTRACTS*

Computerized Information Searching Routes
- Journal articles via MEDLINE
- Journal articles via NURSING & ALLIED HEALTH (CINAHL)
- Journal articles via ERIC
- Journal articles via PSYCINFO

Problem #1

The following is a brief discussion of this problem. In this problem, you are a member of a rehabilitation team working with stroke inpatients. You have noticed that many of your patients have not regained functional use of their arm and several have developed an inferior subluxation of their hemiplegic shoulder. You have decided to conduct a database search on the use of FES. For more information on this problem, please refer to page 114.

Information Searching Strategies for the Use of Functional Electrical Stimulation in the Treatment of Shoulder Subluxation in Stroke Patients (Problem #1)

Computerized Information Searching Routes

Because MEDLINE is one of the main sources of biomedical literature covering a wide selection of clinical journals from many disciplines, this database will be consulted first. Then, a Nursing and Allied Health (CINAHL) search, which covers the nursing and allied health literature, will be conducted. By utilizing these two databases, it is anticipated that we will find the best (most accurate and relevant) articles to answer problem #1.

Journal Articles Via MEDLINE Search

The *MeSH* terms that we chose were **CEREBROVASCULAR DISORDERS** or **HEMIPLEGIA** and **SHOULDER** or **SHOULDER JOINT** and **ELECTRICAL STIMULATION**. (The terms were exploded where appropriate). The following citations were obtained from 1986 to 1989:

1
UI – 87261305
AU – Bohannon RW; Larkin PA; Smith B; Horton MG
TI – Relationship between static muscle strength deficits and spasticity in stroke patients with hemiparesis.
SO – Phys Ther 1987 Jul; 67(7):1068-71

2
UI – 87175907
AU – Bohannon RW; Smith MD
TI – Assessment of strength deficits in eight paretic upper extremity muscle groups of stroke patients with hemiplegia.
SO – Phys Ther 1987 Apr; 67(4):522-5

3
UI – 87123809
AU – Pontinen PJ
TI – Omura's "Bi-Digital O-Ring Test: as a guide to acupuncture treatment.
SO – Acupunct Electrother Res 1986;11(3-4):217-8

4
UI – 87067759
AU – Baker LL; Parker K
TI – Neuromuscular stimulation of the muscles surrounding the shoulder.
SO – Phys Ther 1986 Dec; 66(12):1930-7

5
UI – 87067750
AU – Griffin JW
TI – Hemiplegic shoulder pain.
SO – Phys Ther 1986 Dec; 66(12):1930-7

As you can see, the article by Baker and Parker looks relevant to the topic of interest. The other articles discuss spasticity and the etiology of shoulder pain in the hemiplegic shoulder.

For a more comprehensive literature search, the reader should obtain a list of references that has been published within the last five years.

Journal Articles Via NURSING AND ALLIED HEALTH LITERATURE (CINAHL) Search

The terms used for this search were *ELECTRICAL STIMULATION* and *SHOULDER*. The following citations were obtained from 1986 to 1989:

10/3/1
0059928
Neuromuscular electrical stimulation of the muscles surrounding the shoulder
Baker LL; Parker K
PHYS THER, 1986 Dec; 66(12):1930-7 (24 ref)

10/3/2
0081651
Biofeedback and functional electrical stimulation in stroke rehabilitation
Cozean CD; Pease WS; Hubbell SL
ARCH PHYS MED REHABIL, 1988 Jun; 69(6): 401-5 (15 ref)

10/3/3
0079551
Chronic electrical stimulation for the modification of spasticity in hemiplegic patients
Stefanovska A; Gros N; Vodovni L; Rebersek S; Acimovic-Janezic R
SCAND J REHABIL MED (SUPPL), 1988; No. 17:105-9 (10 ref)

10/3/4
0073513
Relationship between functional electrical stimulation duty cycle and fatigue in wrist extensor muscles of patients with hemiparesis
Patman-Braun R
PHYS THER, 1988 Jan; 68(1): 51-6 (21 ref)

The *NURSING AND ALLIED HEALTH* (CINAHL) search brought up the Baker and Parker article again. The other references (except for article #4 by Patman-Braun, which discusses the application of FES to the wrist muscles) look as if they may contain the necessary information. Upon reading these articles, you discover they do not appear to be appropriate to answer problem #l, as they discuss the application of FES to the lower extremity. So far, the Baker and Parker article seems to be the key reference in the information searching route. The next step is to appraise this paper critically.

The reader should realize that, to ensure that the most accurate and current information is being obtained, a Nursing and Allied Health (CINAHL) search for the last five years should be done.

Methodology Notes for the Critical Appraisal of an Article About a Preventative or Therapeutic Health Intervention for the Use of Functional Electrical Stimulation in the Treatment of Shoulder Subluxation in Stroke Patients (Problem #1)

CITATION: Baker LL and Parker K: Neuromuscular electrical stimulation of the muscles surrounding the shoulder. Phys Ther 66:1930-1937, 1986

The following is an example of how the critically appraised Worksheet (Figure 3-1) found in this chapter can be used:

1. Was The Design Architecture Appropriate?

Yes.

Sixty-three hemiplegic patients with subluxated shoulders of their involved upper extremity were randomly allocated to one of two groups. The experimental group received neuromuscular electrical stimulation (NMES) while the control group received conventional "hemi-slings" or wheelchair arm supports when they were in the sitting or standing position. The patients were not prognostically stratified prior to randomization. NMES is considered to be the same as FES.

Similarity between the NMES and control groups is addressed: time since onset, age, sex, and side of involvement are compared between groups. However, there is no mention of the severity of the disease (that is, the stages of recovery[34]).

We do not know whether the clinicians (who were treating the patients) and the patients were "blind" (unaware of the treatment that the patient was receiving). Lack of "blindness" is a bias that could seriously affect the outcome. For example, it may be that the clinicians in the study may favor NMES and, consequently, would make a greater effort to ensure that the patients improve. Similarly, the patients in the NMES group may feel very fortunate that they are receiving the "wonderful new treatment" and would work very hard to improve their health status.

2. Were All Relevant Health Outcomes Reported?

Can't tell.

The amount of subluxation and its subsequent reduction was determined by x-rays taken of the patients' subluxated hemiplegic shoulders prior to, and at the completion of the study (6 weeks later). Shoulder subluxation was compared with radiographs of the patients' uninvolved shoulders. Stimulation of the posterior deltoid and supraspinatus muscles was used to reduce shoulder subluxation. The radiographs were assessed by two independent observers, only one of whom was "blind."

Muscle fatigue was assessed daily as indicated by a lack of full stimulated reduction of the subluxation, which was estimated by manual palpation. The investigators did not state how manual palpation was done, who measured it and if the assessor was "blind."

Twenty patients, each from the control and study groups, were assessed for the effects of shoulder subluxation on their perceived pain at the shoulder. This assessment was based upon the patients' subjective reports to nursing and physical therapy staff and on the patients' requests for analgesic drugs. We are not sure how these 40 patients were chosen. The severity and duration of these pain episodes were not addressed; pain should have been measured more accurately.

Two patients in the NMES group expressed discomfort at the shoulder joint which appeared to be related to the electrical stimulation. Treatment was suspended for several days until their pain ceased; therapy was then resumed with no further episodes of pain reported. Three-month follow-up radiographs of 11 controls and 13 NMES patients showed no change in the control group subjects. A mean of 1 to 2 mm loss of the subluxation reduction was achieved in the NMES patients. This procedure should have been done for all patients so that we could have an idea of the long-term effects of NMES.

3. Were the Study Patients Recognizably Similar to Your Own?

Yes.

The eligibility criteria stated that all stroke patients had a minimum of 5 mm of shoulder subluxation in their involved upper extremity, as compared with radiographs of their uninvolved extremity. Rancho Los Amigos is a tertiary care facility that does not admit patients during the acute flaccid stage of recovery. The referral pattern was not described. Information was provided on time since onset, age, sex and side of involvement. Exclusion criteria were not defined.

4. Were Both Statistical and Clinical Significance Considered?

Yes – for statistical significance.
No – for clinical significance.

Statistically significant differences (P < .05) in the reduction of subluxation were found between the control and study groups after 6 weeks of NMES and between the pretreatment and posttreatment measurements in the study group. Clinical significance was not addressed.

5. Is the Therapeutic Maneuver Feasible in Your Setting?

Yes.

The therapeutic regimens were well described. Both treatments are available, affordable and sensible. There was no mention of any precautions taken to avoid contamination or co-intervention. In fact, co-intervention may have occurred in the NMES group in the training phase. During this time, the patients used a hemi-sling or wheelchair arm support between and during the treatment sessions. We do not know if the clinicians and the patients were "blind". In this study, it would be difficult to "blind" the therapists for they can actually see who is receiving the NMES (it was on the patients for up to 6 or 7 hours daily). To overcome this, sham NMES could have been used. Compliance was not addressed.

6. Were All Patients who Entered the Study Accounted for in its Conclusion?

Yes.

There was no mention of dropouts, withdrawals or noncompliers; all patients who entered the study were accounted for in its conclusion.

Conclusion

This randomized clinical trial evaluated the effectiveness of NMES versus hemi-slings and wheelchair arm supports in 63 stroke patients with subluxation of their involved shoulder. The results showed that there were statistically significant differences in reduction of subluxation in the study group after 6 weeks of NMES and between the pretreatment and posttreatment measurements in the NMES group. The main limitation of this study is the lack of "blindness." Although the subluxation was significantly reduced in the patients treated with NMES after 6 weeks, we do not know about the long-term effects of the intervention. Having considered all of the methodological criteria used to evaluate the effectiveness of therapy,[22] it appears that FES may be beneficial in treating subluxated shoulders in hemiplogic patients. However, since these are the results of only one study, more research is needed before recommending such an approach. Therefore, it is suggested that other clinical articles on this topic should be obtained and evaluated.

Problem #2

The following description is a synopsis of problem #2. In this problem, you are wondering if your newly diagnosed client with seropositive rheumatoid arthritis should attend a multidisciplinary education program. Since she has two young children and a husband at home, she would prefer to attend these sessions as an outpatient or read pamphlets on the topic rather than being admitted to the hospital. To assist you in deciding what advice you should give this woman with regard to attending this program, you do a computerized search. For a fuller explanation of this problem, please refer to page 115.

Information Searching Strategies for Educating Patients with Rheumatoid Arthritis (Problem #2)

Computerized Information Searching Routes

To find an answer to problem #2, MEDLINE, NURSING AND ALLIED HEALTH (CINAHL) and ERIC (Education Resources Information Center) searches were conducted. These databases were selected because they encompass the biomedical, allied health and nursing and educational literature.

Journal Articles via MEDLINE Search

For this search, the *MeSH* headings that were chosen were **PATIENT EDUCATION** and **ARTHRITIS, RHEUMATOID** and **CLINICAL TRIALS** or **RANDOM ALLOCATION**. The following citations were obtained from 1983 to 1989:

1
UI – 87270121
AU – Gerber L; Furst G; Shulman B; Smith C; Thornton B; Liang M; Cullen K; Stevens MB; Gilbert N
TI – Patient education program to teach energy conservation behaviors to patients with rheumatoid arthritis: a pilot study.
SO – Arch Phys Med Rehabil 1987 Jul; 68(7):442-5

2
UI – 85071567
AU – Parker JC; Singsen BH; Hewett JE; Walker SE; Hazelwood SE; Hall PJ; Holstein DJ; Rodon CM
TI – Educating patients with rheumatoid arthritis: a prospective analysis.
SO – Arch Phys Med Rehabil 1984 Dec; 65(12):771-4

The reference by Gerber et al addresses the issues of teaching energy conservation behaviors only. Although this article is a randomized controlled trial in which patients were allocated to either a workbook group or a traditional occupational therapy group to receive instruction in energy conservation, it is not broad enough to deal with all aspects of the management of rheumatoid arthritis. It would not have sufficient information to answer problem #2. The Parker et al article looks as if it may contain the necessary information.

Journal Articles Via NURSING AND ALLIED HEALTH LITERATURE (CINAHL) Search

For this search we used the headings of **ARTHRITIS, RHEUMATOID** and **PATIENT EDUCATION**. The following references were obtained from 1983 to 1989:

3/3/1
0082997
The effects of patient-practitioner interaction on compliance: a review of the literature and application in rheumatoid arthritis
Feinberg J
PATIENT EDUC COUNS, 1988 Jun; 11(3);171-87 (55 ref)

3/3/2
0080026
Nature and source of information received by primiparas with rheumatoid arthritis on preventative maternal and child care
Conine TA; Carty EA; Wood-Johnson F
CAN J PUBLIC HEALTH, 1987 Nov-Dec; 78(6): 393-7 (28 ref)

3/3/3
0074489
Evaluation of a problem-solving intervention for patients with rheumatoid arthritis
DeVellis BM; Blalock SJ; Hahn PM; DeVillis RF; Hochbaum UM
PATIENT EDUC COUNS, 1988; 11(1): 27-42 (18 ref)

3/3/4
0070122
Patient education program to teach energy conservation behaviors to patients with rheumatoid arthritis; a pilot study
Gerber L; Furst G; Shulman B; Smith C; Thornton B; Liang M; Cullen K; Stevens MB; Gilbert N
ARCH PHYS MED REHABIL, 1987 Jul; 68(7): 442-5 (15 ref)

3/3/5
0062391
A program for improving energy conservation behaviors in adults with rheumatoid arthritis...PRECEDE model for educational diagnosis
Furst GP; Gerber LH; Smith CC; Fisher S; Shulman D
AM J OCCUP THER, 1987 Feb; 41(2): 102-11(16 ref)

3/3/6
0047263
The effects of patient education on patient cognition and disease-related anxiety... rheumatoid arthritis outpatients
Berg CE; Alt KJ; Himmel JK; Judd BJ
PATIENT EDUC COUNS, 1985 Dec; 7(4): 389-94 (16 ref)

3/3/7
0085112
Educating patients with rheumatoid arthritis: a prospective analysis
Parker JC; Singsen BH; Hewett JE; Walker SE; Hazelwood SE; Hall PJ; Holstein DJ; Rodon CM
ARCH PHYS MED REHABIL, 1984 Dec; 65(12): 771-4 (21 ref)

As we can see, this search produced an extensive list of references. The first two articles can be eliminated since the topics discussed in them are too specific and would not contain enough information to answer problem #2. The third article by DeVellis et al is a RCT in which 101 patients with rheumatoid arthritis were allocated to a problem solving intervention group and a control group. Since this paper covers the topic of problem solving only, it would not be broad enough to encompass all of the relevant issues in the management of rheumatoid arthritis (especially for a patient who has been newly diagnosed as we have in problem #2). The Gerber et al article can also be eliminated as it addresses energy conservation behaviors only. The fifth reference by Furst et al, which discusses the PRECEDE model for energy conservation behaviors, is not a randomized controlled trial. The Berg et al paper can also be eliminated as it mainly addresses the issue of anxiety. At this point in the information searching process, it appears that the Parker et al article may provide some of the answers to problem #2.

Journal Articles Via ERIC (Education Resources Information Center) Search

Since this topic deals with educational issues, we decided to do an ERIC search. We used the headings of **RHEUMATOID ARTHRITIS** and **EDUCATION**. When we added the term **PATIENT EDUCATION** to **RHEUMATOID ARTHRITIS**, the search revealed that there were no published articles. The following references were obtained from 1980 to 1989:

7/3/1
EJ359584 HE522923
Development and Application of a Computer Simulation Program to
Enhance the Clinical Problem-Solving Skills of Students.
Boh, Larry E.; and Others
American Journal of Pharmaceutical Education, v51 n3 p253-61
Fall 1987

7/3/2
EJ354937 SP516815
School Problems and Teacher Responsibilities in Juvenile
Rheumatoid Arthritis.
Taylor, Janalee; And Others
Journal of School Health, v57 n5 p186-90
May 1987

7/3/3
EJ267254 HE516034
Impact of Intensive Education and Interaction with Health
Professionals on Patient Instructors.
Riggs, Gail E.; And Others
Journal of Medical Education, v57 n7 p550-56
Jul 1982

7/3/4
EJ229537 AA532080
Rx in the Classroom.
Ladd, Frances T.; And Others
Instructor, v90 n2 p58-59
Sep 1980

By glancing at these citations, it looks as if they do not cover educating patients with regard to the management of rheumatoid arthritis. Thus, the Parker et al article should be obtained and critically appraised.

Methodology Notes for the Critical Appraisal of an Article About a Preventative or Therapeutic Health Intervention for Educating Patients with Rheumatoid Arthritis (Problem #2)

CITATION: Parker JC, Singsen BH, Hewett JE, Walker SE, Hazel-wood SE, Hall PJ, Holstein DJ, Rodon CM: Educating patients with rheumatoid arthritis: a prospective analysis. Arch Phys Med Rehabil 65, 771–774, 1984

The following is a discussion of how to critically appraise this article based on the use of the Critical Appraisal Worksheet (Figure 3-1).

1. Was The Design Architecture Appropriate?

Yes.

Twenty-two men with rheumatoid arthritis (RA) were randomly assigned to either a patient education group, receiving standard inpatient medical care in addition to a formal education program, or to a control group, receiving only the inpatient medical care. Prior to randomization, the subjects were prognostically stratified for functional level (class I, II, or III). The groups could have been stratified for other variables that may have had an impact on the outcomes, such as the type and amount of medications that they were taking and their joint counts. The patients in the groups were similar with regard to age, degree of life stresses, socioeconomic status, educational level and years since onset of RA.

The main bias in this study is the attention bias, which is that the study patients may systematically alter their behavior when they know they are being observed. Also, the health care workers may spend more time with the experimental group and, as a result, they could do better than the control group. As well, the experimental group may do better simply because of the group interaction.

2. Were All Relevant Health Outcomes Reported?

Yes.

Outcome measures were taken prior to, and after, the intervention. There was a follow-up assessment (3 months after the termination of the study) to determine the long-term effects. The instruments used were the Arthritis Knowledge Inventory (AKI), the Arthritis Impact Measurement Scales (AIMS) and the Beck Depression Inventory (BDI). The instruments were pretested for reliability and validity. It may have strengthened the study if the authors had quoted the reliability and validity figures. The outcomes reported were quite comprehensive. We cannot be sure if the outcome assessments were "blind." Other measures such as work status and medications could have been considered.

3. Were The Study Patients Recognizably Similar To Your Own?

No.

This study includes only men; the average age of the study population is 55 years which may be somewhat older than most patients with RA. The study takes place in a tertiary care facility. There were no inclusion criteria other than the patients had to be diagnosed as having RA. The exclusion criteria of previous formal patient education, history of organic brain syndrome, presence of a major psychotic disorder, presence of other uncontrolled medical disorders, presence of a major communicative disorder, illiteracy and patients with American Rheumatism Association functional capacity class IV were well stated. The results are limited to this specific population and cannot be generalized to other RA populations.

4. Were Both Statistical And Clinical Significance Considered?

Yes.

Statistical significance was found. That is, there was a statistically significant increase (P < .001) in knowledge as determined by the AKI, a significant increase (P < .05) in impaired physical activity in the AIMS at post-test and 3 months follow-up and a significant increase (P < .05) in pain in the patient education group than in the control group.

Clinical significance was discussed. Because pain is a multidimensional phenomenon that includes cognitive, emotional and sensory determinants, it can be greatly affected by an individual's mental set. The authors of this article felt that perhaps the educational group experienced increased pain because of certain educational materials that were presented. The pain experience may have been reinterpreted and possibly magnified in these materials; that is, detailed pictures of joints were displayed or concepts of "joint erosion" were used to explain the underlying pathology of RA. Similarly, the concept of "joint protection" to teach lifestyle changes may have inadvertently heightened a sense of vulnerability in some patients. A sensitization may have occurred in which patients assumed too strong a relationship between movement and potential joint damage.

5. Is The Therapeutic Maneuver Feasible In Your Setting?

Can't tell.

Contamination was avoided as patients were assigned to different wards. However, the control group may have acquired helpful tips from the health care workers or other patients chatting with them. Co-intervention may have occurred as there is no mention of the medications that were given to the patients. Perhaps the use of medications accounted for the results. Although standardization of the maneuvers was attempted by providing us with a description of the source of the educational materials, the description of the maneuvers was incomplete. The therapeutic maneuver was not "blind."

6. Were All Patients Who Entered The Study Accounted For In Its Conclusion?

No.

Although 22 patients were selected, complete follow-up and analysis were done on 18 patients. What happened to the other four? Did they drop out? Were they too sick to continue in the study? What were their sociodemographic characteristics? Four out of 22 patients is a sizeable dropout rate. The investigators should have obtained information on these patients because patients who withdraw from a study may differ systematically from those who remain.

Conclusion
This study evaluated the effects of an education program on a stratified randomized sample of 22 men with RA and compared the results with a control group who received standard inpatient medical care. The results were that there was less overall disability in both groups, improved dexterity in both groups, little impact on social role for those in the education group, decreased depression in both groups, a significant increase in knowledge in the education group, a significant increase in physical impairment in the education group, and a significant increase in pain in the education group.

A major limitation of this article is that the results are too specific to this study group and therefore they cannot be generalized to other RA populations. Also, this study is not generalizable to the newly diagnosed RA female patient. Because of the seriousness of the flaws in this study, a search of the earlier literature should be conducted.

Problem #3

The following is a synopsis of problem #3. In this problem, you are a nurse on the maternity ward of a hospital and you have noticed that many of your patients complain of urinary incontinence postpartum. You wonder if an intensive program of pelvic floor muscle exercises would be helpful. You conduct a computerized literature search to find information on this topic. For a fuller description of this problem, please refer to page 116.

Information Searching Strategies for the Use of an Intensive Regime of Pelvic Floor Exercises for Postpartum Patients (Problem #3)

Computerized Information Searching Routes
MEDLINE and Nursing and Allied Literature (CINAHL) searches were conducted. In the MEDLINE search, we used the *MeSH* term of CLINICAL

TRIALS and **RANDOM ALLOCATION** so that we could be assured of obtaining research related articles. The NURSING AND ALLIED HEALTH (CINAHL) database was chosen since it covers the nursing literature. By searching both databases, a more comprehensive search was done.

Journal Articles Via MEDLINE Search

For this search, we used the *MeSH* headings of **PELVIS** and **CLINI-CAL TRIALS** or **RANDOM ALLOCATION**. The following references were retrieved from 1986 to 1989:

```
1
UI  – 88093810
AU  – Sleep J; Grant A
TI  – Pelvic floor exercises in postnatal care.
SO  – Midwifery 1987 Dec;3(4):150-64


2
UI  – 87063698
AU  – Murphy K; Grieg V; Garcia J; Grant A
TI  – Maternal consideration in the use of pelvic examinations in
      labor.
SO  – Midwifery 1986 Jun;2(2):93-7


UI  – 87285985
AU  – Reginald PW; Beard RW; Kooner JS; Mathias CJ; Samarag SU;
      Sutherland IA ;Wadsworth J
TI  – Intravenous dihydroergotamine to relieve pelvic congestion in
      labor.
SO  – Lancet 1987 Aug 15;2(8555) 351-8


4
UI  – 86263025
AU  – Klarskov P; Belving D; Bischoff N; Dorph S; Gerstenberg T;
      Okholm B; Pedersen PH; Tikj O; Wormslev M; Hald T
TI  – Pelvic floor exercise versus surgery for female urinary stress
      incontinence.
SO  – Urol Int 1986;41(2):129-32
```

As can be seen from the example of the citations above, articles 2 and 3 do not address the topic of urinary incontinence. The fourth reference, by Klarskov et al, looks as if it may be worthwhile. Unfortunately, this article could not be obtained at the local health science library since the library does not carry *Urologia Internationalis*. The first article, by Sleep and Grant, is a randomized controlled trial and looks as if it may be relevant to answering problem #3.

Journal Articles Via NURSING AND ALLIED HEALTH LITERATURE (CINAHL) Search

For this search, we used the headings of **PELVIS, RESEARCH, CLINICAL** and **EXERCISE**. The following journal articles were obtained from 1986 to 1989:

3/3/1
0082172
The effect of pelvic floor exercises in the treatment of genuine urinary stress incontinence in women at two hospitals
Henalla SM; Kirwan P; Castledon CM; Hutching CJ; Brocson AJ
BR J OBSTET GYNAECOL, 1988 Jun; 95(6): 602-6 (18 ref)

3/3/2
0078128
Pelvic floor musculature exercises in treatment of anatomical urinary incontinence
Tchou DCH; Adams C; Varner RE; Denton B
PHYS THER, 1988 May; 68(5) 652-5 (18 ref)

3/3/3
0070652
Graded exercises for the pelvic floor muscles in the treatment of urinary incontinence
Laycock J
PHYSIOTHERAPY, 1987 Jul 10: 73(7): 871-3 (12 ref)

3/3/4
0074717
Pelvic floor exercises in postnatal care
Sleep J; Grant A
MIDWIFERY, 1987 Dec; 3(4):150-64 (12 ref)

Although the first three articles cited above appear to address the issues that may answer problem #3, they are not RCTs. The article by Sleep and Grant will be critically appraised next.

Methodology Notes for the Critical Appraisal of an Article About a Preventative or Therapeutic Health Intervention for The Use of an Intensive Regime of Pelvic Floor Exercises For Postpartum Patients (Problem #3)

CITATION: Sleep J and Grant A: Pelvic floor exercises in postnatal care. Midwifery 3:158-164, 1987

The following is a discussion of how to evaluate this article based on the use of the Critical Appraisal Worksheet (Figure 3-1).

1. Was The Design Architecture Appropriate?

Yes.

This is an RCT in which 1800 women, recruited within 24 hours of vaginal delivery, were allocated to follow either a more intensive regime of pelvic floor exercises endorsed by the use of a 4 week exercise diary (experimental group) or receive instructions in pelvic floor exercises (control group).Similarities between the groups are documented: maternal age, parity status, type of delivery, trauma during delivery (such as episiotomy or tear), incontinence during pregnancy, and whether the patients did pelvic exercises during pregnancy, the baby's gestational age and the baby's birth weight. Although the groups were generally similar at entry, more women in the intensive exercise group reported that they had urinary incontinence during pregnancy (32% versus 29%) and did pelvic floor exercises during pregnancy (57% versus 46%). To eliminate these differences, the patients should have been stratified on these variables prior to randomization.

Since the patients could be recognized by the possession of diaries, the clinicians were not "blind." This is a major bias. The health care workers may favor intensive pelvic floor exercises and consequently will give these patients extra encouragement as they want them to do better. Attention bias also exists. This bias states that study patients may systematically alter their behavior when they know that they are being observed. The patients who were instructed to do the pelvic exercises and were asked to fill out the diaries may work extra hard to please the clinicians.

2. Were All Relevant Health Outcomes Reported?

Can't tell.

Outcome measures were taken by community midwives who visited the patients on their tenth postnatal day. At 3 months postpartum, all the women were mailed a standardized questionnaire. This questionnaire sought to obtain the following information: the prevalence and frequency of urinary incontinence, the prevalence and severity of residual perineal pain, the time of resumption of sexual intercourse, the prevalence of dyspareunia, the prevalence of fecal incontinence and the woman's feelings of general well-being. Unfortunately, the investigators did not state whether the questionnaire was pretested for reliability and validity. The outcome assessments were not "blind."

3. Were The Study Patients Recognizably Similar To Your Own?

Yes.

The study was conducted at the maternity unit of a general hospital in England. The eligibility criteria were that every morning, except Sundays, women who had a vaginal delivery in the preceding 24 hours were invited to participate. Women whose babies were stillborn or seriously ill were excluded from the trial.

4. Were Both Statistical And Clinical Significance Considered?

Yes.

The chi square test was used to compare frequencies in the two groups. There were no statistically significant differences in the groups with regard to prevalence and frequency of incontinence. However, there was a statistically significant difference in reduction of perineal pain in the intensive therapy group (chi square for trend = 7.14; $P < 0.01$). Adjustment for exercise use in pregnancy by indirect standardization slightly increased this difference. Also, there was a statistically significant difference in improvement in the women's feelings of general well-being in the intensive program. In particular, fewer women reported feelings of depression (chi square for trend = 5.30; $P < 0.05$).

Clinical significance was somewhat addressed. The authors discussed the fact that perhaps urinary incontinence following vaginal delivery is a result of damage to the innervation of the pelvic floor muscles, rather than stretching of these muscles. Therefore, specific pelvic floor exercises may be of limited value in preventing incontinence. They also discussed the fact that the use of pelvic floor exercises increases perineal muscle tone which may be responsible for reducing perineal pain.

The sample size of 1800 subjects is large enough to show a statistically and clinically important difference.

5. Is The Therapeutic Maneuver Feasible in Your Setting?

Can't tell.

Patients in both groups received initial instruction in pelvic floor exercises. Instruction was offered daily (5 times per week) for the patients in the routine exercise group. Women in the intensive exercise group were individually instructed by a midwife coordinator so that they received an extra exercise session (6 times per week). Prior to discharge, each woman in the intensive therapy group was issued a health diary that she was asked to complete over a 4-week period. Each week the diary described a specific pelvic floor exercise. The women were asked to repeat the exercise as often as they could remember during the day.

The maneuvers are not described well. Approximately 80% of the women were discharged to community midwifery care within 48 hours of delivery where their instructions were continued by either the community midwives or the physiotherapists. Women were discharged from midwifery care 10 to 12 days postpartum. There is no mention as to whether these health care professionals were trained in standardizing the pelvic floor exercise regime. Standardization of the exercises was somewhat attempted by providing the patients who were in the routine exercise group with an explanatory leaflet. However, we cannot be sure of the scope of the materials provided. Compliance was addressed in the intensive therapy group but not in the routine exercise group. Contamination was not avoided as all patients were randomized to the same postnatal ward. Co-intervention may have occurred as there is no mention of other treatments that these patients received during the study. The therapeutic maneuver was not "blind."

6. Were All Patients Who Entered the Study Accounted for in its Conclusion?

Can't tell.

Regardless of the patient's subsequent use of exercises, once a patient entered the study, she was not withdrawn from it. Eighty percent of the women who were eligible for entry during the recruitment phase, entered the trial. About twenty percent of the women who did not enter the study delivered on Sundays, when patients were not being recruited.

Conclusion

This study reports on the results of a RCT in which 1800 women who had a vaginal delivery in the preceding 24 hours were allocated to follow either an intensive regime of pelvic floor exercises (experimental group) or to receive instructions in pelvic floor exercises (control group). This study was designed to evaluate whether either treatment would prevent urinary incontinence. The results indicated that there was no difference in the groups in prevalence and frequency of urinary incontinence, but there was a difference in improvement of severity of perineal pain and feelings of well-being in the intensive therapy group.

The major limitations of this article are that the outcome measures and the treatment maneuvers were not well described. Consequently, we would have difficulty replicating this trial. Also, co-intervention and contamination were not avoided and compliance should have been monitored in both groups. Because of the major biases and concerns in the study, another literature search should be conducted and other articles on this topic found and critically appraised.

Summary of the Information Searching and Critical Appraisal Process

When critically appraising clinical journal articles, the assessment should be based upon at least three articles. In many instances, when it is impossible to find three journal publications on a topic, the results of two articles may be acceptable. However, the searcher must base this judgment upon the quality of the articles and how they measure up to the critical appraisal criteria. Another factor to consider is that the journal articles should be fairly current. The searcher should search for articles that have been published within the last five years. Consideration should be given also to all of the methodological criteria that are used to assess the effectiveness of therapy. In most cases, the conclusion as to whether the therapy does more good than harm is a judgment call.

References

1. Sackett DL, Haynes RB, Tugwell P: Clinical Epidemiology: A Basic Science for Clinical Medicine. Boston, Massachusetts: Little, Brown & Co., Inc., 1985.

2. Domholdt EA, Malone TR: Evaluating research literature: The educated clinician. Phys Ther 65:487-491,1985.

3. Tugwell P, Bennet KJ, Haynes RB, Neufeld V, Sackett DL: A controlled trial of teaching critical appraisal of the medical literature to MD clinical clerks. Clin Res 30:24IA, 1982.

4. Department of Clinical Epidemiology and Biostatistics, McMaster University, Health Sciences Centre: How to read clinical journals: I: Why read them and how to start reading them critically. Can Med Assoc J 124:555-558,1981.

5. Williams R, Baker L, Roberts J: Information searching in health care: A pilot study. Physiotherapy Canada 39:102-109, 1987.

6. Hightower AB: Continuing education in physical therapy. Physther 53: 16-24,1973.

7. Curry L, Putman W: Continuing medical education in Maritime, Canada: The methods physicians use, would prefer and find most effective. Can Med Assoc J 124:563-566, 1981.

8. Knowles M: Self-directed Learning: A Guide for Learners and Teachers. New York, New York: Associated Press, 1975.

9. Henderson V: Preserving the essence of nursing in a technological age. Nursing Times 75:2056-2058, 1979.

10. Hunt J: Indicators for nursing practice: The use of research findings. J Adv Nurs 6 :189-194, 1981.

11. Miller JR, Messenger SR: Obstacles to applying nursing research findings. Am J Nurs 78:632-634, 1978.

12. Bolton B: Teaching research in rehabilitative counseling: Reactions and issues. Rehab Counsel Bull 21:290-296, 1977.

13. Currier DP: Elements of Research in Physical Therapy. Baltimore, Maryland: Williams & Wilkins, 1979.

14. Oyster CK, Hanten WP, Llorens LA: Introduction to Research. A Guide for the Health Science Professional. Philadelphia, Pennsylvania, Lippincott Co., 1987.

15. LoBiondo-Wood G, Haber J: Nursing Research. Critical Appraisal and Utilization. Toronto, Ontario: CV Mosby Co., 1986.

16. Payton OD: Research: The Validation of Clinical Practice. Philadelphia, Pennsylvania: FA Davis Co., 1979.

17. Friedman LM, Furberg CD, DeMets DL: Fundamentals of Clinical Trials. Littleton, Massachusetts: PSG Publishing Co., 1985.

18. Haynes BR, Sackett DL, Tugwell P: Problems in the handling of clinical and research evidence by medical practitioners. Arch Internal Med 143:1971-1975,1983.

19. Department of Clinical Epidemiology and Biostatistics, McMaster University, Health Sciences Centre: How to read clinical journals: II: To learn about a diagnostic test. Can Med Assoc J 124:703-710, 1981.

20. Department of Clinical Epidemiology and Biostatistics, McMaster University, Health Sciences Centre: How to read clinical journals: III: To learn about the clinical course and prognosis of disease. Can Med Assoc J 124:869-872, 1981.

21. Department of Clinical Epidemiology and Biostatistics, McMaster University, Health Sciences Centre: How to read clinical journals: IV: To determine etiology or causation. Can Med Assoc J 124:985-990, 1981.

22. Department of Clinical Epidemiology and Biostatistics, McMaster University, Health Sciences Centre: How to read clinical journals: V: To distinguish useless from even harmful therapy. Can Med Assoc J 124:1156-1162, 1981.

23. Department of Clinical Epidemiology and Biostatistics, McMaster University, Health Sciences Centre: How to read clinical journals: VI: To learn about the quality of clinical care. Can Med Assoc J 130:377-381, 1984.

24. Department of Clinical Epidemiology and Biostatistics, McMaster University, Health Sciences Centre: How to reader clinical journals: VII: To understand an economic evaluation (part A). Can Med Assoc J 130:1428-1432, 1984.

25. Department of Clinical Epidemiology and Biostatistics, McMaster University, Health Sciences Centre: How to read clinical journals: VII: To understand an economic evaluation (part B). Can Med Assoc J 130:1524-1549, 1984.

26. Department of Clinical Epidemiology and Biostatistics, McMaster University, Health Sciences Centre: Worksheet for the critical assessment of an article about a preventative or therapeutic intervention. Unpublished document.

27. Mauser JS, Bahn AK: Epidemiology: An Introductory Text. Philadelphia, Pennsylvania, WB Saunders, 1974.

28. Campbell DT, Stanley JC: Experimental and Quasi-Experimental Designs. 2nd Ed. Chicago, Illinois: Rand McNally, 1966.

29. Brown BW, Hollander M: Statistics: A Biomedical Introduction. New York, New York: John Wiley and Sons, 1977.

30. Feinstein AR: Clinical Biostatistics. St. Louis, Missouri: CV Mosby Co., 1977.

31. Lachin JM: Introduction to sample size determination and power analysis for clinical trials. Controlled Clin Trials 2:93-113, 1981.

32. Altman DG: Statistics and ethics in medical research: III. How large a sample? Br Med J 281:1336-1338, 1980.

33. Gore SM: Assessing clinical trials-trial size. Br Med J 282:1687-1689, 1981.

34. Brunnstrom S: Movement Therapy in Hemiplegia: A Neurophysiological Approach. Hagerstown, Maryland, Harper & Row Publishers Inc, 1970.

Appendix

How to Read Clinical Journals: V
To Distinguish Useful from Useless
Or Even Harmful Therapy

Department of Clinical Epidemiology and Biostatistics
McMaster University Health Sciences Centre

This consecutive series of Clinical Epidemiology rounds is presenting efficient and effective strategies for busy clinicians to use when reading clinical articles. The general rules for reading clinical articles are summarized in Fig. 1. This final round will consider the reading of clinical journals to distinguish useful from useless or even harmful therapy; the guides for doing so are listed in Table 1. The necessity for this distinction is underscored in the following clinical presentations.

A. A 48-year-old executive is found to have an elevated serum cholesterol level at his annual company-sponsored check-up. He has a negative history and a normal physical exam, and his resting electrocardiogram is not remarkable. A low-fat diet and clofibrate are prescribed.
B. The son of a man who underwent gastric freezing for a duodenal ulcer 15 years earlier is also found to have a duodenal ulcer and is given cimetidine.
C. A circumferential ligature is placed in the cervix of a pregnant woman with a history of spontaneous abortion.
D. A man with severe angina pectoris and severe left main-stem coronary artery narrowing undergoes aorta-coronary bypass grafting on a surgical service that previously carried out internal mammary ligations.
E. After 6 months of inpatient therapy for schizophrenia, a woman is discharged with a prescription for imipramine.
F. A child in whom tuberculous meningitis is diagnosed is immediately given streptomycin (plus isoniazid and rifampin).

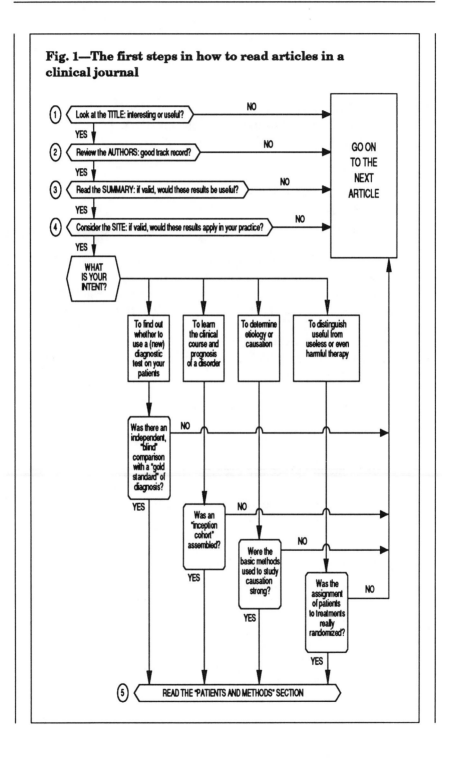

Fig. 1—The first steps in how to read articles in a clinical journal

Table I — A detailed view of readers' guides for intervention studies

1. Was the assignment of patients to treatments really randomized?

2. Were all clinically relavent outcomes reported?

3. Were the study patients recognizably similar to your own?

Validity (Are the results likely to be true?)

Applicability (Are the results likely to be useful?)

4. Were both statistical and clinical signigicance considered?

5. Is the theraputic maneuver feasible in your practice?

6. Were all patients who entered the study accounted for at its conclusion?

G. Two elderly men with transient ischemic attacks are admitted to hospital. One undergoes carotid endarterectomy and the other is begun on a long-term regimen of acetylsalicylic acid.

H. Following a blood pressure rise from 110/70 to 140/90 mm Hg a pregnant woman is given methyldopa.

I. A woman has polyarthritis and a positive test for rheumatoid factor. Indomethacin is prescribed.

J. A child whose 35-dB hearing loss was detected on a preschool exam is booked for tympanotomy and tubal insertion.

These patients have several common features: the central one for this round is that all of them were given treatment intended to prevent (clofibrate in case A), cure (streptomycin in case F) or ameliorate (indomethacin in case I) the disease or illness. Furthermore, all of these interventions were based on the results of basic research into human biology* and behavior, and case series have clearly documented excellent clinical outcomes among patients receiving each of these interventions.

None the less, although we accept some of these treatments as clearly efficacious (that is, we are convinced that they do more good than harm to patients who comply with them), we are doubtful about others and mock the consensus of a former era that embraced gastric freezing and internal mammary ligation. Why is this? One major reason is that we are willing to learn from the experience; the treatments that do more harm than good are, we hope, eventually unmasked. More important, however, is the growth of the attitude, at least in this country, that claims for efficacy need to be backed up by solid evidence, typically from randomized clinical trials, before clinicians will accept them.

This final round will show how to apply some common-sense rules of evidence to the claims for efficacy that appear in clinical journals.

Reader's guides

The rules of scientific evidence for the study of therapy can be summarized into six guides for the busy clinical reader (Table 1). Once again, they constitute "applied common sense" and are designed to maximize the efficiency as well as the accuracy of your clinical reading. These guides are of two sorts as shown in Table 1: the first and last deal with *validity* (Are the results of the study likely to be *true?*) and the second, third and fifth guides deal mostly with *applicability* (Are the results of the study likely to be *useful?*). The fourth guide deals equally with elements of both validity and applicability.

1. *Was the assignment of patients to treatments really randomized ?*

Every patient who entered the study should have had the same *known* probability (typically 50%) of receiving one or the other of

---

*Yes, even internal mammary ligation, for contemporary research had shown that substances injected into the stump of the internal mammary artery could be recovered shortly thereafter from the coronary circulation.[1]

the treatments being compared; thus, assignment to one treatment or another should have been carried out by a system analogous to flipping a coin. It's usually easy to decide whether this was done, for key terms such as "randomized trial" or "random allocation" should appear in the abstract, the Methods section or even the title of such articles.*

As a result, the busy clinical reader has the option of applying this guide rigorously: if you are reading a journal to which you subscribe to "keep up with the clinical literature", rather than searching the clinical literature to decide how to treat a specific patient, discard at once all articles on therapy that are not about randomized trials.

Why such a strict criterion? Why shouldn't clinicians accept the results of trials that are not randomized? A formal explanation for this strict rule is lengthy, but its conclusion is straightforward: random allocation eliminates many of the biases that lead to false results in nonrandomized trials. The pragmatic explanation is brief: we are very much more likely to help our patients and very much less likely to harm them if we institute therapies that have been shown to do more good than harm in proper randomized clinical trials.

Instances in which we have been misled by accepting evidence from nonrandomized trials are numerous and include several of the case presentations that opened this round. For example, clofibrate, as used in case A, was growing in popularity before publication of the randomized clinical trial that showed that it actually increased mortality;[2] the drug was subsequently banned in several countries. Furthermore, it has been estimated that 2500 gastric freezing machines had been used in treating tens of thousands of patients with peptic ulcer — for example, the father in case B — before a randomized trial demonstrated the lack of efficacy of this treatment.[3] Finally, it took a randomized clinical trial in which patients with angina were randomly allocated to undergo or not undergo internal mammary ligation only after their arteries had been surgically exposed to impress on us how often symptomatic improvement can follow placebo medications and procedures.[4]

---

*Beware of "look-alikes" to randomization. For example, some reports describe how patients were assigned "at random" to one therapy or another; often these are *not* randomized trials; the authors of such reports might as well have said that patients were assigned "at the investigators' convenience", "without conscious bias" or even "haphazardly".

In summarizing the situation as it applied to the treatment of rheumatic fever, Bywaters[5] suggested that the proponents of different regimens may be grouped as those with enthusiasm and no controls and those with controls but no enthusiasm. This state of affairs was actually quantified for therapeutic maneuvers in pediatrics by Sinclair,[6] who classified articles on the treatment of respiratory distress syndrome by whether there were controls and whether the authors concluded that therapy was efficacious; his results appear in Table II.

Table II — Relation between alleged therapeutic benefit and the use of control groups*	
Type of study	No. of studies (and % reporting therapeutic success)
Without controls	19 (89)
With controls	18 (50)
Fisher's exact probability = 0.01.	

*Adapted from reference 6.

In summary, then, although the randomized trial can sometimes produce an incorrect conclusion about efficacy (especially, as we shall find out shortly, when it is a small trial), it is by far the best tool currently available for identifying the clinical maneuvers that do more good than harm.

Can we *ever* be confident that a treatment is efficacious in the absence of a randomized trial? Only when traditional therapy is invariably followed by death. Consider case F: Prior to 1946 the outcome of tuberculous meningitis was invariably death. Then, when small amounts of streptomycin became available for use in the United States a few victims treated with this new drug survived.[7] This remarkable result was repeated shortly thereafter in the United Kingdom.[8] Thus, the ability to show, with replication, that patients with a previously universally fatal disease can survive following a new treatment constitutes sufficient evidence, all by itself, for efficacy.

By insisting on evidence from randomized clinical trials you can increase the efficiency with which you read a journal to which you subscribe, for it will lead to early rejection of most of the articles concerned with therapy. The rule requires some modification, however, for reading about a particular patient; often in this instance no proper randomized control trials have ever been published. What should the clinical reader do then?

Two sorts of actions are appropriate when reading about a specific patient. First, the initial literature search should be for any randomized trials that do exist. Second, in the absence of any published randomized clinical trials, clinical readers will have to use the results of subexperimental investigations. Before accepting the conclusions of such studies, clinicians should be satisfied that the improved patient outcomes following therapy are so great that they cannot be explained by one or more biases in the assembly of the study patients or in the assessment or interpretation of their responses to therapy. This second rule is obviously a judgment call and should be tempered by the recollection that this same sort of subexperimental evidence supported the earlier use of clofibrate, internal mammary ligation and gastric freezing. Thus, the situation is a familiar one for clinicians: the need to act in the face of incomplete information. As in similar circumstances this is perhaps best accomplished by considering both the certainty of causation and the consequences of the alternative courses of action (see part IV of this series): Does the patient require *any* intervention? If so, have any of the available interventions been shown to do more good than harm in a randomized trial? If not, which of them is most likely to produce a favourable trade-off between benefit and risk? The following guides may be useful in the critical assessment of proper randomized trials.

2. *Were all clinically relevant outcomes reported?*

Consider Table III, which summarizes the results of an important randomized trial of clofibrate among men with elevated levels of serum cholesterol.[2] Some of the outcomes of therapy appear highly favourable. For example, the serum cholesterol level—a key risk factor for coronary heart disease—fell by almost 10%, providing some biologic evidence for benefit. However, some readers will recognize a claim of therapeutic benefit based on this change in the

Table III — Clinically relevant outcomes in a randomized trial of clofibrate for preventing coronary heart disease*

Variable	Outcome	
	With placebo	With clofibrate
Average change (%) in serum cholesterol level	+1	-9
No. of nonfatal myocardial infarctions/ 1000 men	7.2	5.8
No. of fatal and nonfatal myocardial infarctions/ 1000 men	8.9	7.4
No. of deaths/ 1000 men	5.2	6.2

*Adapted from reference 2.

serum cholesterol level as an example of the "substitution game", in which a risk factor is substituted for its associated clinical outcome,[9] and will want to look further to see whether there were real changes in the occurrence of acute coronary events.

Such evidence is also available in Table III, where we note reductions in the number of nonfatal myocardial infarctions and of all infarctions, both fatal and nonfatal. Thus, the efficacy of clofibrate appears to be supported in this study. However, when we consider all the clinically relevant outcomes, especially from the patient's point of view,[10] we must consider the effects of clofibrate on the quality of life and on total mortality; this is shown with disturbing clarity in line 4 of Table III: the death rate rose with clofibrate therapy, a result that subsequently has profoundly affected both the use and availability of this drug. Thus, because one's judgement about the usefulness of clofibrate or of other agents can depend, in a crucial way, on the clinical outcomes chosen for comparison, readers must be sure that all clinically relevant outcomes are reported.

Furthermore, because clinical disagreement is ubiquitous in medicine,[11] readers should also recognize the necessity for explicit and objective criteria for the clinical outcomes of interest and for the application of these criteria by observers who are "blind" to whether the patient was in the active treatment or control group.

3. *Were the study patients recognizably similar to your own?*

This guide has two elements. First, the study patients must be recognizable; that is, their clinical and sociodemographic status must be described in sufficient detail for you to be able to recognize the similarity between them and your own patients. Second, the study patients must be *similar* to those in your practice. To put it another way, you should ask yourself: Are the patients in this study *so different* from my patients that I could *not* apply the study results in my practice? This requirement goes beyond the fourth general guide for reading clinical journals (the site) to encompass the precise features of individual patients rather than the general features of their referral network. When both recognizability and similarity are satisfied clinical readers will be able to predict with confidence the clinical outcomes to be expected from applying specific therapy to specific patients in their practices.

4. *Were both statistical and clinical significance considered?*

Clinical significance here refers to the *importance* of a difference in clinical outcomes between treated and control patients and is usually described in terms of the *magnitude* of a result. Thus, in Table III we see that the patients taking clofibrate were (6.2–5.2)/5.2 or 19% more likely to die than those randomly assigned to receive a placebo. Such a difference becomes clinically significant when it leads to changes in clinical behaviour;* thus this 19% difference in total mortality is confirmed as being clinically significant when its recognition is followed by a sharp reduction in the frequency if prescribing clofibrate for such patients.

By contrast, *statistical* significance merely tells us whether a difference is likely to be real, not whether it is important or large. More precisely, the statistical significance of a difference is nothing

---

*Although we have defined clinical significance from the clinician's perspective, it could, of course, also be defined from the patient's perspective in terms of "important differences in the quality of life"

more than a statement of the likelihood that this difference is due to chance alone. Thus, if the likelihood is quite low (say, less than 5% or <0.05*) that the 19% difference is total mortality between patients taking clofibrate between patients taking clofibrate and those taking placebo is due to mere chance, we refer to the difference as being statistically significant.

The determinants of clinical significance are therefore the determinants of changes in clinical action; if the results of a study lead you to abandon an old treatment for a new one, the difference in the effects of these treatments is clinically significant. The determinants of statistical significance are not as immediately obvious. Simply stated, the statistical significance of any given result rises (that is, the P value falls) when the number of patients in the study is increased, when the clinical effect of treatment shows less fluctuation from day to day or from patient to patient, and when the measurement of this clinical effect is both accurate and reproducible.

On the basis of the foregoing, the busy reader can use two quick yardsticks for reading therapeutic articles. First, if the difference is statistically significant (P < 0.05), is the difference clinically significant as well? If so, the results are both real and worthy of implementing in clinical practice. Second, if the difference is not statistically significant, are there enough patients to show a clinically significant difference if it should occur? As already discussed, the number of patients in a study is one of the determinants of statistical significance. Thus, if a study population is huge, the difference in clinical outcomes can be statistically significant (real) even if it is clinically trivial (too small to justify a change in clinical behaviour). Conversely, if a study population is too small, even large differences of enormous potential clinical significance may not be statistically significant.† Readers must therefore scrutinize the difference in clinical outcomes in studies whose results are not statistically significant to see whether they are of potential clinical significance. This admonition has received additional weight from the demonstration that most of the recently published randomized trials whose results were not statistically significant had too few patients to show risk reduction of 25% or even 50%.[12]

---

*By convention this likelihood is called the "P value," "alpha," or "the chance of making a type I error," in which we conclude that a difference exists when, if fact, it doesn't.

†This is what is meant by "low power," the "β-error problem" or the "risk of a type II error," in which we conclude that no difference exists when, in fact, it does.

5. *Is the therapeutic maneuver feasible in your practice?*

There are four requirements here. First, the therapeutic maneuver has to be described in sufficient detail for readers to replicate it with precision. Who did what to whom, with what formulation and dose, administered under what circumstance, with what dose adjustments and titrations, with what searches for and responses to side effects and toxicity, for how long and with what clinical criteria for deciding that therapy should be increased, tapered or terminated? Second, the therapeutic maneuver must be clinically and biologically sensible. For example, the dose, route of administration and duration of drug therapy should be consistent with existing knowledge about pharmacokinetics and pharmacodynamics. Similarly, combination of different treatment modalities should make clinical sense.

Third, the therapeutic maneuver has to be available. Readers must be capable of administering it properly and their patients must find it accessible, acceptable and affordable.

Fourth, when reading the description of the maneuver in the published report, readers should note whether the authors avoided two specific biases in its application: *contamination,* in which control patients accidentally receive the experimental treatment, which results in a spurious reduction in the difference in clinical outcomes between the experimental and control groups: and *co-intervention,* when additional diagnostic or therapeutic acts are performed on experimental but not control patients, which results in a spurious increase in the difference in clinical outcomes observed between the experimental and control groups. Once again, it should be apparent that co-intervention is prevented by "binding" both study patients and their clinicians as to who is receiving what treatment.[13]

6. *Were all patients who entered the study accounted for at its conclusion?*

The canny reader will note how many patients entered the study (usually the number of experimental and control patients will be almost identical) and will tally them again at its conclusion to make certain that they correspond. For example, Table IV describes the clinical outcome in 151 patients in a randomized trial of surgical versus medical therapy for bilateral carotid stenosis.[14] Among 79 patients undergoing surgical therapy and 72 patients undergoing medical therapy who were "available for follow-up" (total at the end of the study, 151) a 27% (P = 0.02) reduction in the risk of continued transient ischemic attacks, stroke or death was reported following surgery, a difference that is both clinically and statistically significant. However, closer reading of the report reveals that 167, not 151, patients entered this study and that 16 of them suffered a stroke or died during their initial hospitalization and were excluded from the foregoing analysis. Furthermore, 15 of the 16 patients had been allocated to surgery; 5 of them died and 10 had a stroke during or shortly after surgery. The results of their reintroduction into the final analysis are shown in Table V: the reduction in risk from surgery is now only 16% and no longer statistically significant (P = 0.09).

Table IV — Surgical versus medical therapy in bilateral cartoid stenosis; outcomes among patients "available for follow-up"*

Therapy	Recurrent transient ischemic attacks stroke or death		Total no. of patients
	Yes	No	
Surgical†	43	36	79
Medical	53	19	72

*Adapted from reference 14.
†Risk reduction from surgical treatment: [(53/72) – (43/79)] / (53/72) = 27%.
x^2 = 5.98 and P = 0.02.

Table V — Surgical versus medical therapy in bilateral cartoid stenosis; outcomes among patients randomized*

Therapy	Recurrent transient ischemic attacks stroke or death		Total no. of patients
	Yes	No	
Surgical†	58	36	94
Medical	54	19	73

*Adapted from reference 14.
†Risk reduction from surgical treatment: [(54/73) – (58/94)] / (54/73) = 16%.
x^2 = 2.80 and P = 0.09.

The authors of the foregoing report were careful to include outcome information on all patients who entered their trial, making the construction and interpretation of Table V possible. What can the reader do when the outcomes for missing subjects are not reported? One approach (admittedly conservative and therefore liable to read to the "type II" error) is to arbitrarily assign a bad outcome to all missing members of the group with the most favourable outcomes. If this maneuver fails to shift the statistical or clinical significance of the results across a decision point, the reader can accept the study's conclusions.

Use of These Guides to Reading

The approach to the clinical journal described in this and the other Clinical Epidemiology Rounds in this series is designed for busy clinicians who are striving to keep abreast of important advances in clinical diagnosis, of new insights into the clinical course and prognosis of human illness, of breakthroughs in our understanding of the etiology of disease, and of clinically significant improvements in therapeutics. We clinicians face an awesome task: although already behind in our clinical reading, we are asked to absorb the contents of even more journals each year.

Assuming we will never have more time to read than we do now, and recognizing that critical assessment of the clinical literature is required if we are to do more good than harm to our patients, we have assembled and described a set of common-sense guides for assessing clinical articles. One of the major results of their application is the early rejection of many, indeed most, clinical articles. No doubt in the process in their application some meritorious publications will be cast aside. None the less, we believe that the subset of clinical articles that survive the application of these guides will be the most valid, the most relevant and the most applicable to our clinical practices; thus, they will merit the increased attention that we, in our less encumbered reading, can pay them.

Conclusion

What proportion of papers will satisfy the requirements for both scientific proof and clinical applicability described in the last five Clinical Epidemiology Rounds? Not very many, although there is evidence that matters are improving.* After all, there are only a

*Although cohort studies appear to be losing out to less powerful cross-sectional studies in general medical journals, randomized trials of therapy are on the rise.[15]

handful of ways to do a study properly, but a thousand ways to do it wrong. Moreover, even if a study does satisfy all of these requirements it will not settle a clinical question for all time. At best, it will contribute a small, sometimes only temporary, increment to our ability to relieve suffering and promote health. As well, the results and conclusion of even the soundest studies may provoke sharp and continuing controversy.

The reasons for this slow progress and these disputes are several. First is the possibility that, despite impeccable design and analysis, the study results are flat wrong; this, of course, is the inevitable, although rare, consequence of testing for statistical significance: occasionally results *will* be due to chance alone.

Second, the contemporaneous understanding of human structure and function and mechanisms of disease that led clinical investigators to group certain sorts of patients or responses together may subsequently be shown to have been seriously deficient, negating the results or interpretations of the original study.

Third, a study may be misunderstood or misinterpreted by those who read about it, such as when an explanatory trial designed to answer the question "Can treatment X work under optimal circumstances (e.g., compliant patients, elaborate dose-setting schemes and a restricted set of clinical outcomes)?" is criticized for its inability to answer the management question "Does treatment X do more good than harm under usual clinical circumstances (e.g., all patients, usual dose-setting procedures and the gamut of clinical outcomes)?"[10]

Fourth, controversy can arise over the interpretation of even a valid study when a trade-off must be made between the different results it produces. For example, studies of alternative approaches to managing patients with symptoms of appendicitis have shown that one could minimize the number of deaths from this condition with a liberal policy of operation on all such patients, even those with mild symptoms.[16] On the other hand, if one wanted to minimize the amount of unnecessary surgery, hospital costs or length of convalescence one would adopt a more conservative policy and reserve surgery for patients with severe symptoms. In this instance there are not one but two sharply contrasting "best answers" to the clinical question being posed, and controversy becomes inevitable.

Fifth, study results and interpretations, even those that satisfy the requirements set down in these last five rounds, may meet considerable resistance when they discredit the only clinical approach currently available for managing a condition; clinicians still may elect to do something, even if it is of no demonstrable benefit, rather than nothing. Finally, study results may be rejected, regardless of their merit, if they threaten the prestige or livelihood of their audience.

In summary, this series of rounds is intended to help the serious reader afford time for the proper evaluation of that subset of the clinical literature most likely to yield valid and useful new knowledge. Although it would be naive for us to expect the application of these guides to greatly accelerate the acquisition and clinical application of useful new knowledge, we are confident that their adoption will ensure that whatever momentum is achieved will be forward.

Although the readers' guides have been presented for use in reading the current clinical literature, they have other uses as well. For example, they can aid a literature review, focusing our search and assisting in the identification of the most potentially useful articles. Moreover, in clinical discussions at the bedside or in teaching rounds they can be applied to statements about diagnosis, prognosis, etiology and therapy. Finally, they can be used to organize and present evidence about diagnosis, prognosis, etiology and therapy to students and colleagues.

We welcome feedback about the usefulness of this series for all of these purposes as well as suggestions for their improvement.

We thank our students, house staff and clinical colleagues for their suggestions and criticisms of earlier versions of these ideas.

References

1. Glover RP, Davila JC, Kyle RH, Beard JC Jr, Trout RG, Kitchell JR: Ligation of the internal mammary arteries as a means of increasing blood supply to the myocardium. *J Thorac Cardiovasc Surg* 1957; 34: 661-678
2. Oliver MF, Heady JA, Morris JN, Cooper J: A co-operative trial in the primary prevention of ischaemic heart disease using clofibrate. Report from the Committee of Principal Investigators. *Br Heart J* 1978; 40: 1069-1118
3. Miao LL: Gastric freezing: an example of the evaluation of medical therapy by randomized clinical trials. In Bunker JP, Barnes BA, Mosteller F (eds): *Costs, Risks and Benefits of Therapy,* Oxford U Pr, New York, 1977: 198-211

4. Cobb LA, Thomas GI, Dillard DH, Merendino KA, Bruce RA: An evaluation of internal-mammary-artery ligation by a double blind technique. *N Engl J Med* 1959; 260: 1115-1118
5. Bywaters EG: Treatment of rheumatic fever. *Circulation* 1956; 14: 1153-1158
6. Sinclair JC: Prevention and treatment of the respiratory distress syndrome. *Pediatr Clin North Am* 1966; 13: 711-730
7. Hinshaw HC, Feldman WH, Pfuetze KH: Treatment of tuberculosis with streptomycin: summary of observations on 100 cases. *JAMA* 1946; 132: 778-782
8. Medical Research Council: Streptomycin treatment of tuberculous meningitis. *Lancet* 1948; 1: 582-596
9. Yerushalmy J: On inferring causality from observed associations. In Ingelfinger FJ, Relman AS, Finland M (eds): *Controversy in Internal Medicine,* Saunders, Philadelphia. 1966: 659-668
10. Sackett DL, Gent M: Controversy in counting and attributing events in clinical trials. *N Engl J Med* 1979; 301: 1410-1412
11. Department of Clinical Epidemiology and Biostatistics, McMaster University, Hamilton Ont.: Clinical disagreement: I. How often it occurs and why. *Can Med Assoc J* 1980; 123: 499-504
12. Freiman JA, Chalmers TC, Smith H Jr, Kuebler RR: The importance of beta, the type II error and sample size in the design and interpretation of the randomized control trial. Survey of 71 "negative" trials. *N Engl J Med* 1978; 299: 690-694
13. Sackett DL: Design, measurement and analysis in clinical trials. In Hirsh J, Cade JF, Gallus AS, Schonbaum E (eds): *Platelets, Drugs and Thrombosis: Proceedings of a Symposium held at McMaster University, Hamilton, Ont. October 16-18,* 1972, Karger, Basen, 1975: 219-225
14. Fields WS, Masleniko V, Meyer JS, Hass WK, Remington RD, MacDonald M: Joint study of extracranial arterial occlusion. V. Progress report of prognosis following surgery or nonsurgical treatment for transient ischemic attacks and cervical carotid artery lesions. *JAMA* 1970; 211: 1993–2003
15. Fletcher RH, Fletcher SW: Clinical research in general medical journals. A 30-year perspective. *N Engl J Med* 1979; 301: 180-183
16. Neutra R: Indications for the surgical treatment of suspected acute appendicitis: a cost-effectiveness approach. In Bunker JP, Barnes BA, Mosteller F (eds): *Costs, Risks and Benefits of Surgery,* Oxford U Pr. New York. 1977: 277-307

Glossary of Terms

Bias — Refers to the difference between the true value and that actually obtained due to all causes other than sampling variability.[27]

Blindness — In a "blind" trial, the group allocation is unknown to the observer(s) and the investigator(s). Both the subject(s) and the investigator(s) do not know to which intervention the subject(s) has been assigned. Blindness is an attempt to avoid potential bias.

Clinical Significance — Refers to the importance of a difference in clinical outcomes between treated and control patients that usually is described in terms of the magnitude of a result and that may lead to changes in clinical behavior.[22]

Co-intervention — Refers to the bias that occurs when additional therapeutic and diagnostic acts are performed on the experimental but not the control group.

Compliance — Refers to how well the patients and the health care workers follow the treatment maneuvers.

Contamination — Refers to the bias that occurs when the control group accidentally receives the experimental treatment.

Design Architecture — Refers to the type of research design used in clinical trials.

Randomization — Is a process by which each person or element in a population has an equal chance of being selected to either the experimental group or the control group.

Reliability — Refers to the consistency or constancy of a measuring instrument.

Research — Is the systematic, logical and empirical inquiry into the possible relationships among particular phenomena to produce verifiable knowledge.[15]

Statistical Significance — Refers to whether a difference is likely to be real as opposed to occurring due to chance, and whether it is important or large.[22]

Stratification — Involves distributing any (prognostic) factor that may affect the results of the trial equally among the experimental and the control groups in an effort to minimize its influence on the results.

Type I Error or Alpha Error — This occurs when we conclude that there is a statistically significant difference in the results of the two treatments being evaluated in a research trial when, in fact, there is not.

Type II Error or Beta Error — This occurs when we conclude that there is no statistically significant difference in the results of the two treatments being evaluated in a research trial when, in fact, there is.

Validity — Refers to the determination of whether a measurement instrument actually measures what it is purported to measure.

Index

All references to figures are in italics. All references to tables are denoted by a "t".